# Conversation on the Dung Heap

## Reflections on Job

*Rosemary A. Hubble*

*A Liturgical Press Book*

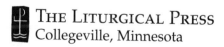
THE LITURGICAL PRESS
Collegeville, Minnesota

Cover design by Greg Becker.

1      2      3      4      5      6      7      8

Library of Congress Cataloging-in-Publication Data

Hubble, Rosemary A., 1938–
    Conversation on the dung heap : reflections on Job / Rosemary A. Hubble.
        p.    cm.
    Includes bibliographical references.
    ISBN 0-8146-2503-7 (alk. paper)
    1. Bible. O.T . Job—Meditations.   2. AIDS (Disease)—Religious aspects—Christianity—Meditations.   I. Title.
BS1415.4.H83   1998
223'.106—dc21                                              98-13342
                                                CIP

*For*
*Caroline, Julie, Christopher*
*and*
*Jackson*

# Contents

# Acknowledgments

I give my thanks to the many people who have helped in the writing of this book, especially to:

My many teachers who have shared their wisdom and knowledge.

Miss MacDonald, headmistress of The Abbey School in England, who, in my childhood, taught the Bible as a living document.

Undergraduate and graduate professors Barry Levis, Hoyt Edge and Arnold Wettstein of Rollins College, Florida, and Jeffrey Kuan and John Endres of the Graduate Theological Union in Berkeley.

Bill Countryman has been not only a teacher and friend but a resource for the title of this book.

The community of The Cathedral Church of Saint Luke in Orlando, where my journey of critiquing, deepening and transforming my faith started.

The people of Good Shepherd, Berkeley for sustaining the process, especially Kathleen Van Sickle, Deacon in Charge, for her egalitarian care of the sometimes unruly sheep of Good Shepherd.

Minda Lucero for her help in editing the early manuscript and my son, Chris, for his astute editorial touch.

My daughter Caroline for her companionship in the journey and the many, many patients, their families, partners and friends who have shared their stories.

# Introduction

Tragedy, catastrophic disease and natural disasters bring upheaval to life, pain and suffering to our souls, even as they compel us to reflect upon the meaning of our lives within the context of a chosen faith tradition. Today, the effects of the Human Immunodeficiency Virus (HIV) upon people can be overwhelming. Women, children and men who face this tragedy, whether personally or professionally, frequently find the meaning gone from life and life itself in chaos.

Since my first experiences, in 1985, with the effects of HIV, I have become aware that in the last breaths of the twentieth century a retrovirus is causing a "massive, dynamic and unstable"[1] global pandemic. Even today, when the new protocols of protease inhibitors appear to be stemming the flood of deaths in the United States, the HIV pandemic marches on relentlessly upon the earth.

The physiological response to the virus not only makes the human body vulnerable to opportunistic disease, but the associated condition, Acquired Immune Deficiency Syndrome (AIDS), exacts an overwhelming and terrifying toll in pain, suffering and death. The challenge of living with HIV is forcing us to critique, deepen and transform the images by which we create meaning for ourselves in relationship with God and others.

My work as a hospice nurse—caring for terminally ill women, children and men, their families, life partners and friends—exposes me to much pain, suffering and death. Frequently there are no acceptable answers to the sickness, pain, grief and the "why me?" of illness and death. Although death is rarely welcomed, most women and men would agree that life eventually must end. As sisters and brothers in life's journey, we can and must let go. However, it has become increasingly difficult for me to accept the global devastation of the HIV pandemic.

The enormous pall this deadly virus has spread across the world exposes our vulnerability, unveils the frailty of life and reveals the depth of sorrow that is part of the intrinsic fabric of human existence. And yet, in the midst of this tragedy, my world-picture has expanded and deepened as I have reflected upon the experiences and stories of women, men and children affected by HIV. I have come to realize the presence of God in the midst of this tragedy.

In this time of the HIV/AIDS pandemic I frequently read *Job* in the Hebrew Bible. The story of the man from Uz has brought hope and an answer to the human question which has been asked in times of trouble throughout the ages. It is the question verbalized by Eliphaz the Temanite and repeated countless times today in this time of AIDS:

> Can a mortal be of use to God?
> Can even the wisest be of service to him? (Job 22:2).

*Job* answers with a resounding "Yes" and shows a God whose arms are spread wide across a universe in pain. This God is willing to meet with me, this God cares for my spirit and enables me to constantly renew my vocation in the world.

The writer of *Job*, Poet Job, proclaims there are no simple answers, no right ways to live and no perfect theology. Poet Job does, however, passionately speak of the pain and suffering which is an innate part of human existence. The story of Job validates the human response to tragedy and reveals a God who cares for the human spirit, always. Therefore, I find *Job* a profound help for spiritual reflection when troubles come.

My reflections have uncovered the similarities between Job's story and our stories, especially in this time of AIDS. Job has become, for me, the person who flings open the door to speak of human tragedy with guts, emotionality and companionship. The biblical text reveals that Job held on to his integrity while he faced the physical, social and emotional devastation inherent to all catastrophic occurrences, including illness.

The reader of *Job* follows Job's journey out of the silence of affliction. She or he will hear the verbalized anger of Job's pain and suffering as he argues against theodicy (a vindication of divine justice in the face of the existence of evil) and retribution theology (punishment or reward based upon actions in this world).

The reader will recognize the crucial role of the three friends from afar. They play an essential part toward the processing of Job's pain and suffering when they sit and converse with Job on a dung heap. The phrase "dung heap"² is reflective of how people throughout the ages have shunned the ill, sick and poor, often to the point of casting them as society's "untouchables." The companionship of Job's friends reminds us of the need each of us has for support in times of trouble.

Ultimately, this achingly honest book about human pain and suffering gives no quick fix, no easy answer, no simple formula for healing humanity's tragedies. But *Job* is a touchstone for women and men to reflect upon as they face the dissonance, disorder, chaos, pain and suffering endemic to any catastrophic disease, and explicitly now, when HIV is devastating our globe. *Job* is a wonderful resource for reflection in times of trouble.

## – 1 –

# Prologue

The petticoats of dawn were flecked with blood as my car pulled to a stop before the home of a forty-year-old woman who had just died from the effects of the Human Immunodeficiency Virus (HIV). A group of friends and observers were gathered outside the iron bars guarding the gateway to the shack she called home. A pathway was made for me as I was recognized as the nurse who had admitted her to Hospice Services two days previously.

Stethoscope in hand I listened for breath in her chest or a heartbeat of life; there was none. I turned to face the three generations of women who had nourished and nursed her in her last few weeks of life. A daughter, a mother and a grandmother stood silently watching, waiting for me to tell them the reality they already knew in their hearts. Yes, she is dead.

As I watched these stoic, poor women accept death, I knew I was also witnessing the painful reality of the spiraling numbers of women claimed by the HIV pandemic. Before my very eyes, I saw the pain, the loss and the suffering innate to this tragedy of our times.

As I hugged them I felt for the mother who had coped with her daughter's death sentence and who had held her as she vomited blood; now tears filled her eyes. Here, the grandmother who had had to reconcile not only the wasting of a young body but also the premature death of her future; her worn and wizened face appeared withered and wan, without outward tears; wasted, she felt, in my cradling arms. And the daughter, who had bathed and diapered her mother as she did her own baby daughter—she clung to me as she burst into a storm of uncontrolled tears and wailing.

In all the chaos brought into this home by loss and grief my eyes rested upon a book on top of the television set. It was a family Bible opened to the third page of *Job*. I read at the top of the page, "Let the stars of its dawn be dark; let it hope for light, but have none" (Job 3:9). I recalled the words at the end of that chapter: "I am not at ease, nor am I quiet; I have no rest; but trouble comes" (Job 3:26).

I am not at ease, nor can I be quiet in this time of AIDS. Now, as I recall that tragic scene, I remember the dawn pushing away the darkness as I had driven up to the home. Light had returned, as it always does. I wondered, "Why had this family turned to *Job* in their time of trouble?"

– 2 –

# Job Has AIDS

Then Satan answered the LORD, "Skin for skin! All that people have they will give to save their lives. But stretch out your hand now and touch his bone and his flesh, and he will curse you to your face" (Job 2:4-5).

*Job* is religious discourse depicting the human response to tragedy. Tragedy takes place within community and, therefore, exists within the language of human conversation and the stories of women and men. *Job* is the story of the man Job not only in conversation with his friends and God but also in dialogue with his faith tradition.

Our observations and interpretations of our life experiences are expressed through language. The search for meaning also takes place this way to be either shared with another in conversation or held within the self. Conversation becomes the metaphor for the activity done through language. Conversation is constantly fed by trace perceptions, requires re-negotiation of meaning, affirms change, lives in uncertainty and relies on story.

## Job and My Journey

In this time of AIDS the stories are numerous and multifaceted. Each of us has her or his own. Gene Robinson reports that whole generations of African tribes have been annihilated by the HIV disease. In Uganda,

> many homes are closed up; some villages are left with a couple of elderly women and a handful of children; the sugar factory has closed for lack of laborers.[3]

I have been touched by many stories of children who are brought into the world as HIV positive, their mothers ignorant of their own HIV status. Due to the stress placed upon the immune system by childbirth, these new mothers soon die. Often the biological fathers are not known. As a result, many of these baby girls and boys lie rejected and without parents in sterile hospital wards until death clutches them as well, into its cold claws.

I have played with a child whose mother died and whose father could no longer walk but wanted to see his children grow up. I have stood by the bed of a Roman Catholic nun as she left her sisters of faith. I have stood by helplessly as a gay man cried while he watched his lover and life partner die, all the while knowing that he, too, will soon die.

I have held the hand of a dying man who as a teenager had visited San Francisco and, unknowingly, had become infected. Later, still asymptomatic, he married his high school sweetheart. But when he was diagnosed with AIDS he was deserted by his wife, friends and family. He died telling me he had seen God.

In the early days of the pandemic, I argued with the church hierarchy that we must respond with compassion to all who are affected by the HIV/AIDS pandemic and not preach judgment, punishment from God (retribution theology) and exclusion in our churches. I have lived with an anger of hopelessness, helplessness, humility, exhaustion. I have questioned God, "Why?" I have learned that anger is appropriate as I face the devastation of suffering:

> they are not recognized in the streets.
> Their skin has shriveled on their bones (Lam 4:8).

As a lifelong member of the Anglican Communion, I accept scripture as an integral part of my faith tradition and a primary source for my spiritual growth. Consequently, in these troubled times I have turned to the quintessential religious text people refer to most in times of need, the Hebrew Testament book of *Job*.

I believe I turn to *Job* in times of tragedy because I, like most women and men, either consciously or subliminally, recognize the very human essence of the man living in Uz called Job. I see his frailty, his fear, his vulnerability, his pain and his suffering. I hear his questioning of God and, ultimately, I recognize his trusting faith in a God who created him. In Job I see myself.

Few people, myself included, when faced with catastrophic loss, fall on their knees and worship God as Job did:

> the LORD gave, and the LORD has taken away; blessed be the name of the LORD (Job 1:21).

Although these words reflect a profound wisdom, few of us have the spiritual maturity to be able to express them with integrity. Even so, I find *Job* to be a companion as I travel a road too often filled with pain and suffering, especially in this time of AIDS. *Job* is for me an ageless touchstone for reflecting upon the painful questions which arise wherever tragedy casts its dark shadow.

## Job's Story

A poetic writer of post-exilic Israel,[4] Poet Job tells the didactic tale of a materially prosperous, religious and good man who loses everything but his life because of a wager between God and Satan:

> Then Satan answered the LORD, "Does Job fear God for nothing?" . . . The LORD said to Satan, "Very well, he is in your power; only spare his life" (Job 1:9, 2:6).

Job's children are killed, his property destroyed and his means of income lost. Satan inflicts "loathsome sores on Job from the sole of his foot to the crown of his head" (Job 2:7).

Job is very, very human in his response to his personal losses, sickness, pain and suffering. He is overwhelmed and in despair as he laments his changed status. Even his wife tells him to curse God and die. In his hopelessness, Job sits among the ashes and rubbish of his community's dung heap.

Presently, he is joined by three men from afar, Eliphaz the Temanite, Bildad the Shuhite and Zophar the Naamathite. The three men do more than just commiserate with Job. They become one with him as they sit in silence together. They become Job's emotional brothers and are exiles with Job on the dung heap.

They all sit for seven days without speaking. Then Job breaks the silence and enters into discourse with these brotherly friends from other lands. The interactive communication, the dialogue cycles which emerge, are the sounding board for Job as he challenges his faith tradition's beliefs about pain and suffering. The brotherly friends, unwittingly, help Job process his pain and suffering.

Even though Job must listen to the diatribe of a fourth friend, he becomes aware of a God who cares for his spirit: "and your care has preserved my spirit" (Job 10:12). Job eventually experiences direct interaction with God (theophany) when God speaks to him from the whirlwind, "Then the LORD answered Job out of the whirlwind" (Job 38:1).

Job's theophany is a personal awakening, which Gerald Janzen describes in this way:

> In a manner which eludes propositional statement, but which works to invite reader participation, both the divine questions to Job and his own questions to God are resolved in a covenanting convergence which implies transformed perspectives on the character of God and on the status and vocation of humankind in the world.[5]

At this point, Poet Job has challenged the Israelite tradition's view of an omnipotent and transcendent God. This new image of God is one Harold Kushner describes as follows:

[God] is limited in what [God] can do by the laws of nature and by evolution of human nature and human moral freedom. I no longer hold God responsible for illness, accidents and natural disasters, because I realize that I gain little and lose much when I blame God for those things.[6]

Women, men and children must now see themselves, as Job came to see himself, as integral parts of the universe working with God to bring order and justice to all. This implies a world-picture greater than the individual. It awakens the self to the other, accepts vulnerability and acknowledges the interdependence of all of creation. The story ends with Job restored to health and well-being, surrounded by his seven sons and three daughters, Jemimah, Keziah and Keren-happuch.

## Job's Illness and HIV/AIDS

Poet Job's plot has Job's illness brought about by a wager between God and Satan. Today's modern, scientific mind finds a number of plausible diagnoses for Job's disease. It is clear from the descriptive passages that he not only had sores or lesions all over his body but that he also experienced severe, generalized malaise and exclusion from his society. The skin lesions limit the diagnosis to yaws, smallpox, plague, psoriasis, syphilis, dermatitis herpetifomis and parasitic infection. The most probable disease, however, is yaws.[7]

Regardless of the diagnosis for Job's illness it is clear not only that Job suffered physically but that he was perceived to be unclean. In the eyes of his society, he became an untouchable. Uncleanliness in antiquity was associated with skin lesions, leprosy, dropsy (full of water), flux (probably venereal disease) and intestinal disorders.[8] Of course, in antiquity, the causative factors for these diseases were unknown.

By contrast, we know that Acquired Immune Deficiency Syndrome (AIDS), is caused by the Human Immunodeficiency Virus (HIV). The HIV was identified in 1983 as the causative factor for AIDS. The virus is classified as a retrovirus because it contains the enzyme, reverse transcriptase. This virus is able to incorporate its genetic material into the host cell's deoxyribonucleic acid (DNA), thereby creating abnormal cells which replicate the virus instead of the normal cell. The mutated cells invade the human body's tissues to create biological chaos. Because the HIV retrovirus has an affinity for the immune system's T-helper lymphocytes (T4 cells), the host's immune system is greatly jeopardized and the infected person becomes highly vulnerable to disease.

There is a broad spectrum of HIV-related diseases and conditions which can range from a diagnosis of HIV+ without symptoms, to mild complaints of general malaise, to serious, life-threatening infections. A diagnosis of AIDS is made when a person who is HIV+ develops one or more of a specific group of diseases or conditions identified by the Centers for Disease Control (CDC) as criteria for a diagnosis of AIDS.

Opportunistic infection (OI) is the name given to a broad spectrum of diseases which affect a person with AIDS and are usually the cause of death. These infections are commonly caused by organisms in the environment which rarely make a healthy person sick. However, a person may be very ill from HIV without meeting the CDC criteria for a diagnosis of AIDS.

Although it would satisfy our modern, scientific minds to make a specific diagnosis for Job's condition, it is not important. What is important is to acknowledge the similarities of Job's situation with that of any woman, man or child experiencing one of life's great afflictions and, specifically, AIDS.

The presenting factors of Job's condition, as described by the observer, Elihu, reflect my observations of a person sick with end-stage AIDS, for:

> They are also chastened with pain upon their beds,
> and with continual strife in their bones,
> so that their lives loathe bread,
> and their appetites dainty food.
> Their flesh is so wasted away that it cannot be seen;
> and their bones, once invisible, now stick out
> (Job 33:19-21).

A person with AIDS will recognize in the words of Job her or his own experience and say with him:

> And now my soul is poured out within me;
>     days of affliction have taken hold of me.
> The night racks my bones,
>     and the pain that gnaws me takes no rest . . .
> My inward parts are in turmoil, and are never still; . . .
> My skin turns black and falls from me,
>     and my bones burn with heat (Job 30:16-17, 27, 30).

Job and his modern companion with AIDS, who also finds no rest and faces a prognosis of death, echo this lament throughout the universe:

> so I am allotted months of emptiness,
>     and nights of misery are apportioned to me.
> When I lie down I say, "When shall I rise?"
>     But the night is long,
>     and I am full of tossing until dawn.
> My flesh is clothed with worms and dirt;
>     my skin hardens, then breaks out again.
> My days are swifter than a weaver's shuttle,
>     and come to their end without hope (Job 7:3-6).

A person living with AIDS will experience extremes of general malaise, wasting, anorexia, debilitation and the ravages of raging opportunistic diseases running unchecked throughout a body without an immune system. The multiple lesions and sores God allowed Satan to afflict on Job "from the soles of his feet to the crown of his head" (Job 2:7) can be likened to the Kaposi Sarcoma tumors found throughout the body tissues of people infected with HIV and in the devastation of psoriasis.

"And he has shriveled me up" (Job 16:8) is the quintessential description for the wasting of AIDS. "My skin hardens, then breaks out again" (Job 7:5) parallels the eternal struggle to maintain skin integrity without decubitus. "My flesh is clothed with worms and dirt" (Job 7:5) symbolizes the fear many people have about the disease and their inability to touch a person with AIDS.

"My face is red with weeping, and deep darkness is on my eyelids" (Job 16:16) describes the universal mourning associated with the HIV pandemic. And, finally, Job's ostracism—sitting amongst the ashes on a dung heap—is symbolic of not only destruction but alienation from society which becomes emblematic of today's victimization of women, men and children who are HIV+.

In this time of AIDS, when a retrovirus is turning modern reality upside-down, "Job is no longer a man; he is humanity!"[9] And humanity has AIDS. Job has become my friend in my journey of travail during the HIV pandemic. Job has helped me to recognize my stories in his story and has revealed evolving, transitional traces of an unfinished revelation.

# Reflection

The rain fell gently as I stood with my back to the Washington Memorial and looked toward the Reflecting Pool and the Lincoln Memorial. At my feet thousands of pieces of three-by-six-foot oblongs of white cloth made a collage of the HIV/AIDS pandemic. Each one of these small, grave-size memorials was a stark reminder of the power a microscopic organism has to create dissonance, disorder, chaos, pain and suffering in our lives.

On each one of these stark panels loving fingers had crafted symbols of a loved human life. A baby bottle and pacifier, sequins and a Drag Queen outfit, a high school Prom Queen photograph, tender poems of remembrance and love, a leather jacket and motorbike symbols, a patchwork of teddy bears. On and on, row after row, block after block, death upon death they stretched. What stories of human pain, suffering and grief were told in that kaleidoscope of color and design.

Those same diligent fingers which had crafted and stitched to make the Names Quilt Memorial had reached out to touch, nurture and nurse another human being until she or he had died. How many there were, how silently and slowly we walked, child, mother, lover, friend, partner, father, companion, caregiver. I stood there silently remembering all who have no quilt except in the hearts of those who knew them and in the heart of God.

Later, as darkness fell, I stood with friends by the Reflecting Pool for a candlelight vigil. The fragile light from our eight candles flickered and mingled with thousands of other gentle lights. We quietly formed a circle to read, slowly, one by one, the names of the children, women and men we have known who have died from HIV. Often the pages were just passed around the circle because we wept too many tears to read. We finished reading the names and started to read the Prayers for the Dead. Strangers came up to us and asked if a loved one's name could be added, and then they joined our prayer circle.

The circle of grief becomes bigger and bigger.

----------

Through my reflections on *Job* in a time of AIDS I have realized there are no fixed answers for the human story when tragedy occurs but that women, children and men have many stories to share.

The stories are unique to each one of us but each will have recognizable traces of the universal struggle to find meaning in a time when disease brings tragedy into the human experience.

The ancient text *Job* is one such story. Its language is interactive and, therefore, it draws the reader into dialogue with Job because Job's conversations with his friends abound in descriptive passages of the human experience with disease, pain and suffering.

A woman or a man devastated by the HIV/AIDS pandemic will recognize her or his experiences in Job's experiences. At other times, the language of *Job* resonates with our deepest feelings.

# – 3 –

# Chaos

Job said:
  "Let the day perish in which I was born,
    and the night that said,
    'A man-child is conceived.'
  Let that day be darkness!
    May God above not seek it,
    or light shine on it.
  Let gloom and deep darkness claim it.
    Let clouds settle upon it;
    let the blackness of the day terrify it" (Job 3:2-5).

The tragedy of disease brings pain, suffering, disorder, dissonance and chaos into life. Dis-ease, dissonance and chaos entered Job's life and have now entered twentieth-century life by the invasion of the HIV retrovirus. Poet Job uses complex literary structure, various literary genres, dramatic and verbal irony and word play to project an enduring picture of humanity's travail in a time of tragedy. Two thousand years later, this powerful text still has the ability to resonate with us in times of tragedy.

All biblical texts are embodied in rhetorical discourse which inevitably reflects historical and cultural perspectives from the time of the writing. *Job* is no exception. *Job* reflects the multiple hidden threads of Poet Job's world-picture.

It is not difficult to imagine the Hebrew poet of *Job* reflecting upon his own people's stories. These stories would be full of their history, their religion and recent experiences. The poet would recognize in the stories the universal human experience of tragedy.

The gifted writer of *Job* crafts a text to project the chaos, dissonance, and dis-ease tragedy brings to human living. The text's chaotic literary structure, along with its heavy reliance on irony, projects a subliminal ethos of dis-ease, dissonance and chaos. Poet Job's frequent references to darkness, silence and battle with primordial beasts de-constructs both the Israelite's and our own more stable world-pictures. Poet Job's literary style is thus a forceful tool which creates an ethos for Job's story and ours today when faced with tragedy.

**Structure: Chaos**

Poet Job uses dialogue cycles as a fundamental literary structure of *Job*. The poet starts Job's story with dialogues between God and Satan which take place in a polytheistic court. Job experiences great personal loss and physical illness as a result of the wager made between God and Satan. Immediately the plot causes unease for women and men who believe in a monotheistic religion and an omnipotent God. Note, too, that these stage-setting dialogues are completely unknown to Job and the other characters of the book. The reader, by contrast, is aware of them, and so, again, dissonance exists for her or him from the very beginning.

Poet Job continues the plot to have Job destitute and an outcast of his society sitting amongst the ashes on a dung heap. Here Job is joined in his desolate state by three men from afar. They all sit in silence for seven days. As an outcast the righteous man, Job, presents an uncomfortable picture.

The literary structure of dialogue resumes when Job breaks the silence with a lament which is followed by the first round of speeches to form the first dialogue cycle (Job 4–14). This round of speeches introduces a pattern of conversation between Job and his friends. The first to respond to Job, Eliphaz presents Israel's orthodox justification for human suffering. Job answers Eliphaz and is followed by Bildad. Job again speaks, Zophar responds and Job closes the first cycle of conversation. A second round of conversation follows the same pattern (Job 15–21).

During these opening conversation cycles, Job's friends try to be of help by espousing the traditional explanation for the tragedies which bring dissonance, disorder, chaos, pain and suffering into human lives. Unfortunately, by the end of the first cycle, Job is already questioning their explanations. Conflict arises. Dis-ease is felt. For Job does not agree with their justification for pain and suffering. Indeed, he later demands that God appear face to face in "court" (Job 23:4) to defend a world in which innocent suffering exists.

Job's friends try to explain his ill fortune as divine punishment for wrongdoing, i.e., a retribution theology. Eliphaz self-righteously states: "those who plow iniquity and sow trouble reap the same" (Job 4:8), "human beings are born to trouble" (Job 5:7), and "The wicked writhe in pain" (Job 15:20).

Bildad continues this theme when he says, "If your children sinned against him, he delivered them into the power of their transgression," (Job 8:4) and "God will not reject a blameless person, nor take the hand of evildoers" (Job 8:20). Zophar repeats this theme: "the exulting of the wicked is short, and the joy of the godless is but for a moment" (Job 20:5). But Job has done no wrong!

The third dialogue cycle (Job 22–27) becomes disjointed as the established pattern of speeches breaks down. The cycle starts as before, Eliphaz answers Job and Job responds but then the arguments of the friends appear to be spoken by Job. Scholars disagree about who speaks what next. There is a short speech from Bildad, Job speaks an oath of integrity and then there is a final speech generally credited to Zophar. Chaos appears to have entered the very structure of the text and disease continues to be felt.

Through this structural chaos, Poet Job powerfully projects Job's confusion. Job is reflecting upon his experiences, his faith tradition and what he has heard from his brotherly friends. Pain and suffering make no sense in a world Job believes God created to be good.

The text continues in an aura of chaos with Job speaking a poem on the search for wisdom. The poem, however, is without the characteristic Joban complaints. More confusion. This poem on the search for wisdom is full of Job's observations of the human search for wisdom in the material of the world; it creates a change in pace from the dialogues of expounded theology:

> Surely there is a mine for silver,
>   and a place for gold to be refined.
> Iron is taken out of the earth,
>   and copper is smelted from ore. . . .
> They put their hand to the flinty rock,
>   and overturn mountains by the roots (Job 28:1-2, 9).

and continues:

> But where shall wisdom be found?
>   And where is the place of understanding? . . .
> The deep says, "It is not in me,"
>   and the sea says, "It is not with me" (Job 28:12, 14).

Many commentators view this poem as an intrusion, a "superfluous prelude" or an "orthodox afterthought"[10] and believe its form "differs radically from its surroundings."[11] The poem, however, is a pivotal part of the book. It can be seen as a continuation of Poet Job's reflections and, therefore, as connected with the preceding chapters.

Poet Job is, as usual, deliberate in the words he chooses in closing the poem and the first half of the book with this verse:

> And he said to humankind,
> "Truly, the fear of the Lord, that is wisdom;
>   and to depart from evil is understanding" (Job 28:28).

The poet reminds the reader that the first words we heard about Job were that he was "one who feared God and turned away from evil" (Job 1:1). Closure of Job's struggle with his pain and suffering has occurred. But there are no answers. Disease continues. Chaos reigns.

At this point, Poet Job has Job rejecting the traditional wisdom as expounded by his friends. This is not a comfortable projection for the reader. Job is realizing that wisdom is not found through piety, as his tradition had taught. Wisdom, Job has realized, is beyond human skill to obtain but is discovered in the "very process of creation"[12] and living.

The second half of the book starts with a renewal of Job's complaints (Job 29–30). "The night racks my bones" (Job 30:17), "they abhor me, they keep aloof" (Job 30:10) and "I have become like dust and ashes" (Job 30:19). Job recognizes his present position as an ill man, an untouchable, cast onto the dung heap with the rubbish of society. Job has believed that, "there is no one to deliver" him (Job 10:7) and now poignantly expresses his total loss of hope "I cry to you and you do not answer me" (Job 30:20). His pain and suffering are palpable and make for discomfort.

Poet Job concludes Job's final complaint with an oath of purity in which he denies impurity, dishonesty, adultery, failure of hospitality, avarice, idolatry, vindictiveness and hypocrisy.[13] Job has been a good man. Job has done no wrong! To hear Job again lamenting after the conclusion of "the search for wisdom" poem produces yet more dissonance.

"The words of Job are ended" (Job 31:40) trumpets forth. But a fourth friend, Elihu, must have the last word. Elihu enters the story as a self-appointed arbitrator. The introduction of a totally *new* "friend" produces more disruption and inner turmoil within the reader. Why is he here? Hasn't everything been said?

Elihu's point is that Job's request for God to appear before a human court is unreasonable. Elihu insists on the transcendent and unapproachable position of God. If Job suffers then it is because he has done wrong and God is punishing him.

Elihu's speech is couched in legal rhetoric; his concern is for legal process rather than Job's plight. He continues the theme of justification by way of correct religious behavior and piety. He tells Job:

> And if they are bound in fetters
>    and caught in the cords of affliction,
> then he declares to them their work
>    and their transgressions, that they are behaving arrogantly.
> He opens their ears to instruction,
>    and commands that they return from iniquity (Job 36:8-10).

Elihu's speech closes with a diatribe of orthodox theodicy against the innocent Job who is in total revolt. Dissonance, disorder, disillusionment and despair dominate as the structure has dissolved into chaos.

The climax of the book occurs when, unexpectedly, Yahweh comes to Job out of a whirlwind (a theophany). Poet Job's God does not deny that innocent suffering exists in the world. But, instead of giving comfort, instead of affirming Job's goodness or even revealing the truth of the heavenly wager, Yahweh addresses Job with a multitude of rhetorical questions about creation. These questions point to the awesome nature of the cosmos—but they are not very helpful. They are certainly not the defense Job expected.

Job acknowledges that he is indeed of small account. He then lapses into silence. Whereupon Yahweh challenges Job to "gird up your loins like a man" (Job 40:7) and prove he is the equal to Yahweh. Without waiting for Job's response, Yahweh acknowledges that evil exists and declares the awesome nature of the work needed to maintain order in creation. Discomfort is felt if a supposedly omnipotent God has problems keeping the creation in order.

Job, at this point, can do nothing but acknowledge the inbreaking of God into human existence and says for all humanity:

> "I had heard of you by the hearing of the ear,
>    but now my eye sees you" (Job 42:5).

Job is aware that a covenanting convergence has occurred which "implies transformed perspectives on the character of God and on the status and vocation of humankind in the world."[14]

The poet's use of prose for the epilogue is discordant after multiple chapters in beautiful verse. The epilogue tells of Job seeking forgiveness for his friends from the Lord (Job 42:7-9) and a materialistic, mortal, finite world going on after loss and suffering have occurred. Not quite the expected ending.

The epilogue, in a limited text, speaks of humankind's tremendous endurance to go on with living and to survive tragedy. It also appears to support retribution theology. The retribution theology theme, when juxtaposed with Job's covenantal convergence, leaves the reader at the end of the story in a subliminal ethos of dichotomy, dissonance and conflict.

## Irony: Dis-ease and Dissonance

The tragedy-induced ethos of dis-ease and dissonance in *Job* relies heavily upon Poet Job's use of irony. Irony is an "evasive form of expression."[15] Dramatic and verbal, explicit and implicit, subtle and not so subtle irony in Poet Job's literary style make a deliberate contrast between apparent and intended meaning, between pretense and reality, between what should happen and what does happen. This irony soaks the text in dis-ease and dissonance. The irony-induced dissonance is the cradle for Job's struggle.

Dramatic irony begins immediately in *Job*. The prose prologue establishes the plot whereby the reader is given knowledge of the wager between God and Satan which is unknown to Job and friends. The subsequent dialogue cycles, Job's soliloquy and the poem on the quest for wisdom are permeated by the poet's skillful verbal references to the prologue.

It is not difficult to imagine Poet Job reflecting upon the tales heard during the Babylonian exile and making a choice to use them in his story about human pain and suffering. Most scholars agree that well-known texts from the Ancient Near

East—namely *The Babylonian Theodicy* and *Man and His God*[16]—have elements similar to Job's story. In *The Babylonian Theodicy* we read, "I am finished. Anguish has come upon me," and, "My strength is weakened, my prosperity has ended."[17] *Man and His God* echoes humanity's lament, "The malignant sickness-demon bath[es] in my body . . . (My god) how long will you neglect me, leave me unprotected?"[18]

Both *The Babylonian Theodicy* and *Man and His God* confirm the commonality of poetic response to human suffering throughout the ages. Perhaps these very texts formed the springboard for Poet Job to create one of humanity's greatest rhetorical discourses on pain and suffering.

The prologue of *Job* introduces a folklore hero, a righteous man named Job, who is experiencing great suffering and loss as a result of a wager between God and Satan over the issue of disinterested piety:

> Then Satan answered the LORD, "Does Job fear God for nothing?" . . . "You have blessed the work of his hands . . . But stretch out your hand now, and touch all that he has, and he will curse you to your face" (Job 1:9-11).

In this initial scene Job is not a Hebrew man but "a man in the land of Uz" (Job 1:1). God is portrayed as the supreme lord of a polytheistic court who is assessing the yearly portent for humanity.

Poet Job's God allows Satan to inflict loathsome sores on Job. Not quite the picture we expect of the Israelite's monotheistic religion and an omnipotent God. Dissonance and dis-ease, therefore, are immediately established with the first chapter of the book through the poet's use of dramatic irony.

The polytheistic court establishes for the story of Job an ethos of dis-ease and dissonance. This atmosphere continues when Job, stripped of everything that gave meaning to his life, is joined by three friends (Job 2:11). Ironically, these are not Israelite men but men from afar.[19] These three consoling[20] friends spend seven days with Job in silence amongst the ashes on a dung heap. Through the silence of the dung heap the world is returned to pre-creation chaos. There are no words. Gone is God's creative power (Gen 1:1).

Poet Job, having created a story steeped in dramatic irony, imbues the dialogue cycles with verbal irony. The poet does this through the interplay of texts. Job's words will be spoken by one of the friends to project a totally opposite meaning from the one Job intended. Scenes or expressions used by one of the friends will be subtly changed by Job to create a different feeling and/or interpretation. In this way Poet Job continuously reveals the differences between the players and establishes an ethos of dis-ease and dissonance for Job's story.

The manipulation of known Hebrew texts is another form of verbal irony in *Job*. Poet Job's parody of Psalm 8 is one of the most ironic passages of the Bible. The psalmist, in Psalm 8, speaks of the awesome sense of majesty within the cosmos and of the loftiness of the creator in contrast to human frailty and fallibility. Nonetheless, the psalmist indicates this frail human is made in the image of God and called into a higher vocation with the creator, "Yet you have made them little lower than God" (Psalm 8:5). Poet Job, on the other hand, has Job mocking this idea, claiming that God is a "watcher of humanity" (Job 7:20) and that humanity is God's target and a burden. This is verbal irony at its best.

Irony, however, is most explicit in the divine speeches. In the eyes of Job's friends, God should not speak with Job. Yet God does. The inappropriate happens. Religious propriety is subverted. Dramatic irony startles the reader and dis-ease is felt.

Irony continues through the rhetorical questions Yahweh poses to Job because they are prefaced by the remark, "Tell me, if you have understanding" (Job 38:4).[21] Yet they are questions which are clearly unanswerable by a human being. Even today, with all the advances in modern scientific knowledge, many of the questions Yahweh asks Job are still unanswerable.

Finally, if the rhetorical questions God asks in the theophany are perceived as literary irony, then they are not only genuine questions directed at humanity's role in creation but also questions posed by God about God.[22] Thus, by the pervasive use of dramatic and verbal irony, Poet Job has created an ethos of chaos, dissonance, dis-ease and dichotomy from beginning to end.

## De-construction: Beast, Monster and Virus

A central axis of chaos is a crucial aspect of *Job*. It appears not only in the story but in both its literary form and conceptual frame. The literary form through which Poet Job sets up an ethos of chaos, dissonance, disorder and dichotomy has been discussed above. We will now turn to the conceptual frames Poet Job de-constructs in *Job*.

The disintegration of Job's life as a result of the wager between God and Satan is reflected in the words of Poet Job as the poet de-constructs the Israelite world-picture. The scene of Job and his friends sitting without words for seven days provides a stark realization of the metaphorical return to the ancient idea of primordial watery chaos from which God created the cosmos through the power of words:

> while a wind from God swept over the face of the waters.
> Then God said . . . (Gen 1:2-3).

Now, in the story of Job, the cosmos is without words or form. All order is lost. Job and his friends, sitting amidst the ashes, are returned to the primordial silence from which God moved and spoke to create the universe in seven days.

The central axis of the return of the cosmos to primordial chaos reflects upon the creation account of Genesis 1:1–2:4a which was added to the Yahwist narrative (Gen 2:4b–2:25) by the Priestly writers. It is generally understood that both creation stories have Mesopotamian influences. The Yahwist creation narrative is dependent upon topographical features: "the Lord God formed man from the dust of the ground" (Gen 2:7); it puts man in a garden where rivers flowed and plants grew.

The Priestly narrative, on the other hand, stresses a structured cosmology to depict the world created by the word of God (Gen 1:1–2:3).[23] Poet Job de-constructs this creation narrative with the contrasting lack of words between Job and his friends as they sit in silence on the ash heap. In the silence there is no God and no order. Only primordial chaos exists.

In the Priestly myth God's words create a cosmos with meaning and justice. In this cosmos, humankind, created on earth, develops a world-picture in which human beings are created in the image of God to be God's partner in the continuing re-creation of the cosmos. The Priestly myth's world-picture enabled the Israelites to express their experiences of living, to reflect upon life, to create meaning for life and to speak of God in metaphorical language.

This myth proclaims a world in which the dawn heralds re-creation each day. Darkness and evil are continuously defeated by word and light. The daily and yearly cycles of the natural world signify the ongoing procreation of God's world in seven days. This is a world Job knew to be created from primordial silence by the metaphor of word: "Then God said, 'Let there be light'" (Gen 1:3). And, this is the world returned to chaos by the silence of the ash heap.[24]

The world of meaning which is de-constructed in *Job* is shaped by another mythic pattern, the Baal cycle of battle, victory, kingship, judgment and (re)creation.[25] The analogy of a mythic God in primordial struggle with the creatures of chaos, Leviathan and Behemoth, is used extensively by Poet Job.

The struggle is epitomized in Job's first lament when Job risks arousing the beast of chaos, Leviathan (Job 3:8). Job feels this primordial beast has ravaged his life and turned it upside-down. In the divine speeches even God talks about the unruliness of these beasts. The images Poet Job creates of Leviathan and Behemoth and a world returned to primordial chaos are easily transferred to HIV as it de-constructs our world-pictures today.

## Reflection: Critique, Deepen and Transform

At the time Poet Job wrote *Job,* he and the people of Israel were trying to cope with the pain and suffering of their memories of exile. The poet turned to his religious traditions for help. This is a crucial point. Today, we look to *Job* to help critique, deepen and transform our concept of God in a time of AIDS. We build upon the ancient faith traditions of our mothers and fathers of antiquity to reshape our world of meaning.

The dating of *Job* as a sophisticated literary product ranges from the tenth to the fourth century B.C.E. Most evidence points to a post-exilic era. Gerald Janzen, in his commentary on *Job,* adopts the position that the book was written as the people Israel struggled with the existential tension between their experience of an historical upheaval and their religious tradition.[26] Quoting from two historians of religion, Thorkild Jacobsen and Frank Moore Cross, Janzen agrees with other commentators that *Job* must be located within the history of the religions of the Near East.

Janzen traces the development of the Joban metaphors for God by following Jacobsen as the latter uncovers their history in the previous millennia. Jacobsen establishes that in the ethos of Near Eastern religions the metaphors for the gods in the fourth millennium B.C.E. were "powers immanent in the phenomena of nature, powers willing to come to specific form as the phenomena."[27]

Jacobsen states that third millennium B.C.E. gods transcended nature and society as royal, divine figures. Children, women and men were created to be slaves to serve these gods. By the second millennium B.C.E., gods, at times, were viewed as "personal" deities who stood in direct relationship with the human social order. This view of religion led to an anthropocentric religious world-picture.[28]

Cross, according to Janzen, picks up where Jacobsen leaves off and connects the religion of Israel's ancestors with the second millennium B.C.E. anthropocentric religions of the Near

East. The Priestly traditionalists and the editor(s) of the Deu-
teronomic history gave final form to the epic traditions of early
Israel and their God. These are the stories of Israel in the land
in covenant with Yahweh and make up the Hebrew Bible from
Genesis to Second Kings.[29] The Hebrew religious belief in a
God of reward and punishment (retribution theology) has its
origins in these texts.

The religious traditions embodied in the early books of the
Hebrew Bible were part of Job's world-picture. Janzen quotes
Cross as arguing that the metaphors of God in these texts had
become inadequate because they "suppressed the ambiguities of
history."[30] Cross further claims the significance of *Job* is Poet
Job's criticism of the religious tradition through de-construction
of myths and the use of irony to establish a disjunction from
the "ancient religion."[31] But whereas Cross finds disjunction in
*Job*, Janzen argues that "critique, deepening and even transfor-
mation are taking place"[32] within the continuity of a religious
tradition.

In the tragedy of the HIV/AIDS pandemic where dissonance,
disorder, chaos, pain and suffering permeate our lives, the universal applicability of *Job* is very plausible. The modern reader of
*Job* who lives within the ethos of her or his religious traditions
will turn to *Job* as a known religious discourse for reflection.

The complex literary structure, various literary genres, irony,
word-play and plot powerfully reflect the modern reader's feelings in a time of AIDS. Women and men today are challenged
to subvert their static concepts of God; we are invited to critique, deepen and transform our known religious discourses
that they may become useful tools in times of tragedy.

# Reflection

Early one morning the phone rang, disturbing the security of my sleep. I was needed to attend the death of a young woman in her early twenties. As I hurriedly dressed I remembered how I had admitted her to the hospice program only a few weeks before. I remembered how her mother had expressed her daughter's wish to die at home. I remembered the young woman's thinness, her withdrawal from the conversation and how distressed and ill-at-ease the mother was as we talked about her daughter's diagnosis and prognosis. Waiting, perhaps, for me to show signs of rejection or dis-ease.

As I drove quickly along the empty freeways and down the deserted streets to the woman's home, the headlights of the car made a beacon of light around me. But all else was dark as death. As I stopped the car, the radio announced a storm watch for the area. Stepping from my car I was grabbed by a gust of wind; I watched tree branches tossing high above my head, lost pieces of paper flitted through the air and dark clouds covered the moon and stars. In the safety of my car and the narrow beam of my vision I had been unaware that a storm was brewing.

On entering the home I realized that an emotional storm was in progress. I found the mother huddled on the bed, cradling her daughter while a pet poodle nuzzled her mistress, whining softly. The mother sobbed hysterically, begging not to be separated from her only child. I sat on the bed with her. The wind howled outside, turning garbage cans upside-down and rolling them errantly down the deserted street.

The rains came and I listened to the stories of a mother and daughter whose lives were woven together in love. I heard how this only child had brought joy to the mother's life until the HIV virus had stolen their dreams and turned their lives into chaos. I heard of their struggle to get adequate medical care. I heard of their fear of telling her diagnosis to friends and relatives. Their sense of helplessness, hopelessness, humility and exhaustion resonated with mine.

As she talked and I listened, the mother gradually let go of her daughter and held the poodle in her arms, gently stroking her, soothing her as we continued to talk about her daughter's life and the changes a diagnosis of HIV+ had made in their lives. She spoke of how her daughter used the knowledge of her diagnosis to face the mystery which surrounds life and living. She shared how she had stripped away her masks, how she had been willing to risk becoming an authentic and self-actualized young woman.

Above the crashing sounds of the rain cruelly lashing the windows, the mother told how she and her daughter had drawn strength from their Christian faith tradition and from exploration of feminist wisdom literature and new age beliefs. They had come to realize that life was sacred, that they shared a communal solidarity and compassion. They had experienced an intensified awareness of the simple things of life and a willingness to live each day for the hours and moments given to them.

Finally the storm ceased to rage and representatives from the funeral home arrived. The mother and I stood on the steps as her daughter's body was driven away. Dawn had come, the sky was so bright and blue, the air fresh and clean. I drove away listening to a Bach concerto on the radio. I knew I had faced my own mortality that night.

On reaching the end of the street I passed the mother as she took the dog for a brisk morning walk down the storm-cleansed streets. Her life was continuing with the open wound of her daughter's death now a part of her. The echoes of the dissonance, distress, dis-ease and chaos caused by the HIV/AIDS pandemic would remain with her and me forever.

The memory of the mother walking remains with me.

———

Today, women and men turn to *Job* as the archetypal religious rhetorical discourse to reflect upon when pain and suffering are experienced.

*Job* reveals to us the implicit and explicit dissonance, dis-ease and chaos of our own lives when tragedy comes.

The dissonance of our lives in this time of AIDS is palpable through the words, structure, de-construction of myth and use of irony in *Job*. We realize that Leviathan and Behemoth and the silence of Job and his friends serve as symbols for the chaos brought into life by a retrovirus.

Throughout the biblical story, Job remains totally unaware of the wager between God and Satan. What profound questions arise for a person with HIV/AIDS who has been financially dev-astated, lost countless friends and family to the HIV/AIDS pan-demic and now faces her or his own physical illness:

"Is there something I don't know?" she or he may wonder.

"Is God just?"

"Is God playing with me?"

"Is life only a game of one-upmanship?"

Throughout *Job* the established Israelite tradition of mono-theism is challenged by polytheism. Is there only one God, really?

God allows Satan to cause the loss of everything which gave Job's life meaning. The question, therefore, arises: "Is God omnipotent?" Job had done no wrong. Yet he suffers great loss. Can this be retribution from God or are there other forces at work in our lives? This is not a case of retribution theology, in which an omnipotent God rewards and punishes.

The breakdown in the dialogue cycles, the introduction of an uncharacteristic poem in the mouth of Job and a realization that Job has subverted traditional religious practice add to our feelings of uneasiness as we read *Job*. Again we are reminded of the uneasiness felt in a time of AIDS.

The uncomfortable dichotomy continues to be experienced as we face the ironic truth that *Job* does not have the ultimate answer to pain and suffering in a world that God saw as "very good" (Gen 1:31).

The universality of Job's experiences is humanity's story and we recognize it in this time of AIDS.

We are challenged to critique, deepen and transform our faith traditions and to seek viable metaphors for God.

# – 4 –
# Why Job?

Then God said, "Let there be light"; and there was light.
And there was evening and there was morning, the first day.
God saw everything that he had made, and indeed, it was
very good. And there was evening and there was morning,
the sixth day.

Thus the heavens and the earth were finished, and all
their multitude. And on the seventh day God finished the
work that he had done, and he rested on the seventh day
from all the work that he had done
(Genesis 1:3, 5, 31; 2:1-2).

The "paradoxical themes, heroic setting and uncomfortable
challenges"[33] of *Job* evoke the universality of humanity's search
for viable metaphors of God when dissonance, disorder and
chaos enter the world through the experiences of personal
tragedy. These tragedies challenge our accepted world-pictures
through which we create meaning in relationship to others and
to God. The metaphors and models for the concept of God are
crucial to our world-pictures. In the tragedy of the HIV pandemic, these models are challenged in a world devastated by a
malicious microbe.

Women and men of the Judeo-Christian tradition when con-
fronted by the pain and suffering of the catastrophic pandemic
of our times, often turn to *Job*, as witnessed by the story at the

beginning of this book. Why do people turn to *Job*? How can such an ancient, semitic text be of help to people of the twentieth-century, whose world-pictures are influenced by transcontinental, instant communication and E-mail?

The answer depends upon understanding the differences and similarities between the world-picture of the writer of *Job* and ours. More precisely, it depends upon admitting the universality of humanity's need to name the holy and the experience of human pain and suffering throughout history.

Job is recognized as a man living in the same ecological world as we do. By asking our questions, Job speaks for all of humanity. Job plunges to the depths of his spirituality. Job searches to find language that can express his experience of the God who can be present with Job in his time of pain and suffering.

*Job* tells a story of seeking a relationship with the divine. Poet Job explores a sacred creativity combining cognitive reflection, religious discourse and life experiences. This takes place "in community," as evidenced by his brotherly friends' company. Poet Job recognizes the vulnerability implicit to this process. *Job* requires us to acknowledge the axioms that life is terminal, hard and humbling.

*Job* reminds us that we must respond to the world's pain and suffering. *Job*, ultimately, asks us to accept a God-centered (theocentric) world-picture without didactic form or answers. In this world-picture God is present, always.

### World-Picture: Concept, Metaphor and Model

A world-picture is made up of conceptual images or mental pictures of self in relationship with the world and a higher being/God. We acquire a world-picture as children, "through informal and tacit process. We never learn it explicitly, but inherit it from culture."[34] Along the way each world-picture will be influenced and changed by experiences unique to each individual.

An integral part of a person's world-picture is her or his spirituality. Georgianne Cowan says, "Spirit comes into matter only through the vehicle of our humanness."[35] Spirit is a fundamental force of living and is shaped or created by attempts to form as comprehensive and coherent a picture of self in relationship to a higher being, the holy, God. Spirit drives and feeds our spirituality. Spirit is the creative force of ultimate values and meanings which guide living.[36]

The concept of the holy, therefore, is central to a person's world-picture and living. As concepts frequently are metaphors, it is metaphor which shapes a person's world-picture. The values and meaning of life, a person's spirituality, are, in turn, shaped by these metaphors. Throughout the history of religious experience, the metaphors for the concept of God have become the models for God in specific traditions and cultures.

Metaphors and models for God are rarely learned through didactic instruction but are acquired through an informal and tacit process. Frequently they are based upon human family and/or social power structures. Unfortunately, the metaphors and models for God are, therefore, often authoritarian, abusive and restrictive. Consequently, they have little spiritual power and fail in a time of crisis. Job experienced this failure two and a half thousand years ago, just as a person affected by HIV finds an absence of helpful models in today's established religions.

Frequently, the language of metaphor and model will be culture specific but as the ancient text of *Job* proves a specific cultural text can acquire universal usage. This is both a blessing and a bane. The blessing lies in recognizing in Job's story the universality of our stories; and the bane exists when the cultural ethos, metaphors and models of an ancient story are inappropriately projected onto another culture and time.

Any human world-picture will be expressed through language and will reflect an understanding of the person's world. Language is the human method for creativity, cognitive reflection and communication with others using an agreed upon system of signs and symbols. Language expresses recognition of things and people. We think in it, tell our stories and learn through it. Language expresses not only our experiences but the search for meaning in the acts of living.

In the process of forming a world-picture the human imagination will struggle to express through language concepts which have no tangible reality, e.g., God, love, truth, Satan and AIDS.[37] We recognize these concepts in our lives, are touched by them but acknowledge the inadequacy of language to describe them. At these times we turn to our known world and use metaphors to enable us to speak of these concepts. Metaphor, therefore, is the foundation for religious language.[38]

Aristotle defined metaphor as "giving the thing a name that belongs to something else."[39] For example, the concept of "God" is often articulated using the easily recognizable verbal sign "father." The image of the human concept "father" is then reformed by implicit comparison or analogy to describe "God." The human picture of "father" then becomes the identity of the concept "God."

Models are metaphors which have staying power in a culture. Cultural models are the crucible for early childhood world-pictures and become implicit to our meaning of life as we grow into adulthood. Unfortunately, cultural models of the holy frequently approach the status of concepts, and God "is" the metaphor.[40] Father is God, God is a father. Similarly, HIV/AIDS is enemy, invader, the master of molecular life, alien, contaminator and maker of vulnerability.

Religious models can lose their effectiveness when the experiences of life do not fit the model or when the model becomes oppressive or negative for us. At such times, women and men can critique, deepen and transform their known religious discourses to develop new metaphors which have greater staying power and effectiveness.

The new metaphors then become models and help in future times of trouble. In his time of trouble, Poet Job reflected upon his world-picture and created new metaphors for the concept of God.

## Job's World-Picture

Poet Job's and our world-pictures are expressed through cultural language and metaphor, model and myth which are specific to an historical time and place. Poet Job formed his world-picture from a conceptual understanding of the universe which was very different from ours today.

The poet drew not only from the Hebrew religious tradition and ancient cosmogonists' mythological imagery, but also from astute observation of the natural world. Graphic representation of the Hebrew world showed an earth with lines stretched upon it, bases sunk, cornerstones laid (Job 38:5-6); the clouds were its garments (Job 38:9). Thick darkness was the world's swaddling band (Job 38:9). Sheol, "the land of gloom and chaos, where light is like darkness" (Job 10:22), was very real for Job.

The firmament above the earth was the storehouse of snow and hail and where "the waterskins of the heavens" (Job 38:37) were tilted "to bring rain on a land where no one lives" (Job 38:26). The waters above the firmament were contained within two concentric domes. The heavenly seat of the Divinity rested above the domes.

Poet Job saw a universe thoroughly alive, a world less a static being than a moving event, less an ordered organism in repose than a process taking place before the eyes of children, women and men. The waters of the sea were shut in with doors so that the proud waves would be stopped (Job 38:8,11). Job's earth is populated with living, breeding, and dying animals and birds.

The firmament of the sky above the earth was peopled with Orion, the Bear and Mazzaroth. The great beast, Behemoth, prowled the earth, unafraid and causing chaos. The sea monster, Leviathan, lived freely in the deeps of the sea, feared by all, for:

> No one is so fierce as to dare to stir it up.
>   Who can stand before it?
> Who can confront it and be safe? (Job 41:10-11).

## Our World Picture

Our present world-picture, on the other hand, draws extensively from epistemological knowledge which tends to be staid, solid and stationary to create the mythological language of myth and metaphor for twentieth-century reality. This is a picture of an evolutionary universe in which virus, bacteria and syndrome bring devastation and need to be held back. Newtonian and quantum physics explain what we see from our vantage point on the edge of the Milky Way Galaxy.

In this world-picture it is acknowledged that "in the beginning there was chaos!"[41] The cosmos is made up of microscopic particles of matter, "a straight materialization—a creation—of matter from the energy of the primeval bang,"[42] to form planets which are "globes of matter, much smaller than stars."[43] The stars are "balls of gas, tenuous and hot on the outside, dense and hotter on the inside."[44] Galaxies were described by the nineteenth-century German philosopher, Immanuel Kant, as "island universes."[45]

If Poet Job were writing today he would be part of a culture whose world-picture has been dominated by two major vocabularies. One is the inherited Romantic view which informs the concept of the self and, therefore, the holy, with attributes of passion and soul. This leads toward dedication and a strong sense of purpose. The other, twentieth-century's Modernist world-picture, emphasizes ability to reason, logic, usefulness, rationalization, predictability, honesty and individualism. These two vocabularies have influenced our inherited models of God.

However, as the twentieth century ends, both Romantic and Modernist pictures about self are falling into disuse and a "postmodern" picture of self in relationship with the other and God is evolving.[46] The postmodern world-picture is a result of social saturation through a multiplicity of experiences. These experiences occur because we now live in a global village of great and rapid technological change where the foreigner is now a neighbor. Dilemmas of identity ensue and dislocation of self occurs in relationship to God and our neighbors.

In the postmodern world, a person exists in a continuous state of construction and reconstruction. Established cultural norms are subverted, reflexive questioning and irony exist in a pluralistic culture without a specific center. Change, loss, pain and suffering occur constantly. The postmodern world is frequently an uncomfortable place to be. But it is also a place of wanderings, connections, nuance, traces, ambiguity, variety and opportunity.

### Job's Names for the Holy

Women, men and children use language to identify the holy as "god," "goddess" and, for the Judeo-Christian world, "God." These words are the symbols for the concept of the ultimate being, the holy in religious traditions. But the very nature of the Ultimate defies definition. Even "ultimate" and "being" are metaphors. Symbols and signs are inadequate; silence is the appropriate response. However, in human frailty and vulnerability, metaphors and models are created for God.

Poet Job names God Yahweh, El, Eloah and El Shaddai. This variety of names for God reveals humanity's unending search to find language for the concept of God. It appears that Poet Job reflected upon all his culture's religious experiences to reform his image of the holy and find a viable model for God. His example can help us in a time of AIDS.

Poet Job lived at a time when the Hebrew culture's world-picture incorporated the traditional personal name for God, Yahweh. This concept of God was based on the second millennium B.C.E. concept of personal deities. The origin of the name Yahweh is uncertain, but it probably derives from the Hebrew verb "to be" as used in God's response to Moses' question of God's identity: "I am who I am" (Exod 3:14).

Yahweh was seen to be a covenantal God, a person-like being, involved with Israel's history, the cause of all things and present everywhere:

> Whatever the LORD pleases he does,
>   in heaven and on earth,
>   in the seas and all deeps (Psalm 135:6).

Therefore, it was believed that a God who controlled history must also control and order the forces of nature—including those which cause human pain and suffering.[47]

The anthropic model of the holy led to retribution theology, expounded so diligently by Job's friends. But the belief that trouble, pain and suffering came into the world by God's hand because women and men had acted against God's will became a poor model for Job who believed he had done no wrong.

So Poet Job recalls the older, fourth-millennium B.C.E. names of the gods/powers immanent in nature and the cosmos: El, Eloah and El Shaddai. Found throughout *Job,* these names stem from the Canaanite myths in which the gods were seen to be intimately involved in all of the cosmos.

Poet Job reaches back into a world-picture of gods active in the cosmos and where the chaos of human travail was brought about by the primordial beast Behemoth, the sea monster Leviathan or the storm god Baal. These metaphors enhance his concept of God. Throughout *Job* this creation centered world-picture is present both overtly and subliminally, juxtaposed with the traditional Hebrew covenantal concept of a more human-like God.

The incorporation of the mythic patterns and gods into a Hebrew text are perhaps indicative of a people weaving known fourth-millennium B.C.E. polytheistic world-pictures into their second-millennium B.C.E. monotheistic world-picture.

In *Job,* it appears that Poet Job is questioning the established but newer monotheistic covenantal theology of retribution and self-interest righteousness. At the same time, he seems to argue for the experiential metaphors for the holy which are central to the older immanent, cosmological religions.

The covenantal God of the Hebrew people had perhaps become too anthropic for Poet Job. The poet saw human pain and suffering in the world and realized that retribution theology only added to humanity's pain. He sought a way to reveal God continuing in loving relationship with people instead of condemning a creation that he originally saw as "very good."

## Our Names for the Holy

Today's ethos creates a dominant spirituality in which ultimate being is sought exclusively in the material order. Thus, the holy is defined as science, the superstar, royalty and "stuff." The light of God becomes scientific discovery and "God" an obtainable material thing or being. Legalism and rationality rule. But this prevalent model of the holy not only denies the transcendent—it fails in times of trouble.

In a world restricted to the material, holy transcendence gives way to scientific discovery and rational explanation. The place in our lives for God as the higher being is usurped by individualism.[48] The center of a person's world-picture easily succumbs to consumerism, economic need and individualism.

Fortunately many children, women and men continue to practice a faith centered upon the nonmaterialistic holy of the Judeo-Christian tradition. Unfortunately, the dominant model of this holy usually portrays the omnipotent, transcendent God of retribution theology.

It has surprised me how often in my hospice work a woman or man will express an understanding of God as this "God of retribution." It has been my observation that when life is coming to an end, inner fears of "badness" arise. There appears to be an archetypal rationale that bad things happen only because of something done which has displeased the gods or God.

When we are healthy, most of us can dispel these thoughts of retribution theology, but when death is near they seem to haunt us. Although postmodern culture rejects strong religious affiliation, it is my observation that much of today's culture has its subliminal roots in retribution theology.

I believe that if Poet Job were writing today, he would question the present cultural religious models of God. As he did two thousand years ago, he would have to assess their viability to support children, women and men as they face the pain and suffering of this twentieth-century tragedy, the HIV/AIDS pandemic. To do this Poet Job would turn and look at how the concept of God is played out in the theology of the time and place.

### Theology: Humanity Speaks of God

In the process of responding to the challenges of life and to gain a better understanding of their relationship with God, all people seek intellectual clarity for the nature of God. This is theology. The theology of the Hebrew people is generally accepted to be contained within the covenantal and historical books of the Bible.

*Job*, on the other hand, is placed within the Wisdom texts of the Bible. These texts reflect upon the everyday, the ordinary and the universal, which is less exciting, perhaps, but more relevant to the everyday life of most people. Consequently, a Wisdom text like *Job* is a tool for doing new theology in a time of trouble. But it must be remembered that both the covenantal/historical and the Wisdom traditions influence the theology of *Job*.

Theological interpretations of *Job* vary greatly. Some interpreters claim the book proves divine justice in the face of the existence of evil. Some claim it shows God's indifference to human suffering. Others will point to the theology of retribution enunciated by the friends to justify the equation "suffering = sin." Ridiculing the renowned patience of Job, secularism claims that his rebellious dialogues are justification for agnosticism.

On the other hand, some interpreters claim God to be a friend of the sufferer, the "source but not guarantor of the well-being of humans."[49] For others, God is a God who needs human assistance to keep chaos at bay.[50] A cosmological view of *Job* may even profess Yahweh as sustaining a world hostile to human life and, consequently, the metaphor of humanity as king of the cosmos is shattered.[51]

More recent interpreters are claiming that the Wisdom heritage innate to *Job* has been silenced by Western dogmatic and systematic theology. These interpreters lift up the anthropological and cosmological foci of the Wisdom corpus of the Hebrew Bible. The anthropocentric focus emphasizes the common human experience while it minimizes the God of Israelite faith. This view, however, continues to perpetuate an anthropocentric world view and, potentially, to support secularism and/or atheism.

The wisdom literature's cosmological view as expressed in *Job* culminates in a theophany. This supports a holistic theological understanding of a cosmic, theocentric reality constantly being (re)created day by day, year by year. A theocentric understanding of reality is strongly influenced by reflection upon experience, awe, and bewilderment. It also recognizes the unpredictable power of God to in-break into the present, even as it realizes God's eternal care for the spirits of all women, children and men.

The literary structure of *Job* enables the multiple interpretations outlined above. Women and men today are challenged to live a life of faith within the tension of multiple interpretations. The reader of *Job* must question her or his own cultural metaphors and models of God and, when necessary, create new ones.

The women and men who read *Job* today learn that living with multiple interpretations requires an acceptance of vulnerability and that there are no easy answers to the dissonance, disease, chaos, pain and suffering tragedy brings. Living in an ethos of tension, ambiguity and vulnerability allows for the gift of knowing God in times of trouble.

# Reflection

The sky tipped buckets of water through the floodgates of the watery firmament onto the hard macadam of a cluttered Californian suburban street. I made my way through the deluge from the dry safety of my car into the chaos of another life touched by death. My knock on the door went unanswered.

Carefully I opened the door to be assailed by the sounds of pain and disorder, "Don't touch me!" "We must change you," "I can't take this pain anymore, God where are you? Damn it! where is he?" Quickly I introduced myself, gave the suffering woman on the bed a loading dose of liquid morphine and proceeded to assist her three daughters to finish her personal care.

Quiet and order were restored. After a brief introduction to the principles of pain control, symptom management and "Nursing 101," I left the home with a memory of the patient lying on her bed with a stuffed toy bear comfortably supporting her head, her three daughters sharing their plans for the days ahead. The rain had stopped and streams of water rushed their way into the concrete conduit passageways out to the Bay. As I drove away the wind-driven storm clouds raced above me draping the hills with their nurturing mist.

Time passed and I had the privilege of learning the conceptual images which gave meaning to the life of a woman dying in a time of AIDS. She shared her life experiences as she came to terms with a disease contracted, in her case, through a blood transfusion. Her hopes and fears for her family's future were explored. Her pain and symptoms were controlled and her cries of pain became less. I learned Damn-It[52] was the name of her stuffed bear. She said, "This way I can swear without offending God."

One day I arrived to find two of the daughters sitting on the curb of that cluttered street in suburban California. Inside their mother was signing her will. I joined them curbside to comfort them in silence. As we sat, I noticed that where the macadam of the blacktop met the concrete of the curb a river of moss sprinkled with tiny plants existed. Somehow, despite all the brutality of the pounding traffic, this street life survived. As we talked about the fortitude of nature the daughters grasped their reality.

A few days later AIDS stole another life. The daughters gently bathed their mother for the last time. The time waiting for the funeral home people was spent revealing the meaning of a life. One daughter took a book she had given to her mother twenty years before and slowly read, through her tears, the words she had chosen then to express a mother's role, the meaning of her mother's life to her and her love for the life which gave her birth.

The book was placed in the mother's cold hands. Another daughter jumped up and grabbed an uneaten, favorite candy bar from the bedside table and flung it on the bed; then she kissed her mother and gently placed the candy bar with the book. A framed picture of a grandchild holding the family cat was added. Damn-It the bear joined them with the last apple from her fruit tree. The objects of a life were gathered into the cold, dead hands which had nurtured and loved a family. Hands banded at the wrists with favorite bracelets.

The funeral home people came and gathered the remnants of a life into the cold plastic of the tomb. But no one could deny her the treasures which went with her to the grave. Left behind were the streams of life. The children stood in the rain and watched her go. I left with the pictures of their lives embedded in my heart. Beneath our feet the river of moss existed, nurtured by the life-giving waters from above.

As I drove away, I realized that I had experienced a ritual celebrating the joy of a life lived fully within the ethos of a twentieth-century community. Before me had appeared the images of a life. These images formed a picture created not only by words but also in action and in silence cradled within the creation.

The images of this world-picture I will not forget.

---

In the dissonance, disorder, chaos, pain and suffering experienced in the HIV/AIDS pandemic many women and men frequently find their world-pictures no longer help them cope with this twentieth-century tragedy.

It is difficult to step out of the chaos this virus has brought to our world and objectively look at how an ancient text can help re-image a world-picture of self, the world and God.

*Job* can help us to create viable world-pictures in a time of AIDS.

Metaphor and models drawn from the world around us can enable us to speak of our painful experiences.

*Job* challenges and encourages us to move from our traditional pragmatic and scientific world-picture, where God is held in a box and a virus is the enemy, into a space where experiential epiphany can take place.

Poet Job lived in the same ecological system as today and drew extensively from observation of this world. It is important to remember that however different the world-picture Poet Job created may appear to us today, it is the same world of nature in which we live. We can, therefore, recognize it as we weave our life stories together and seek a viable world-picture of self, of God and our world in a time of AIDS.

# – 5 –

# Sit with Job

There was once a man in the land of Uz whose name was
Job. That man was blameless and upright, one who feared
God and turned away from evil (Job 1:1).

They sat with him on the ground seven days and seven
nights, and no one spoke a word to him, for they saw that
his suffering was very great (Job 2:13).

Every child who is born into this temporal world will at
some time experience a loss of health, an important relationship, material possessions, and, the ultimate loss which comes
to all of us: death. Dissonance, discord, chaos, pain and suffering will, therefore, be experienced, both personally and empa-
thetically, by everyone who lives on this planet Earth. The
inevitable question "Why?" echoes throughout the universe.
And at these times of loss, both religious and not so religious
people turn to Job.

Dissonance, discord and chaos have been discussed in the
previous chapters. Now it is time to turn to the recurrent question of pain and suffering. Many people turn to the Hebrew text,
*Job*, in the midst of the HIV/AIDS pandemic because in Job's story
they see their own experiences of pain and suffering. Women and
men recognize in Job and his friends the eternal human response
when catastrophic disease enters human existence:

> They sat with him on the ground seven days and seven
> nights, and no one spoke a word to him, for they saw that
> his suffering was very great (Job 2:13).

After the silence, a verbal outpouring of pain and suffering
takes place as Job directs his anger at God.

## Who Is Job?

Who is this man named Job? Poet Job chose to create a man
easily recognized as a prototype of a person accepted by society as
good. Therefore, the prose prologue immediately identifies Job as
the wealthy man living in the land of Uz who is "blameless and
upright" (Job 1:1) with a wife, children and property.

Job is a man who religiously practices the pragmatic piety of
his faith tradition not only for himself but for his children:

> And when the feast days had run their course, Job would
> send and sanctify them, and he would rise early in the morn-
> ing and offer burnt offerings according to the number of
> them all; for Job said, "It may be that my children have
> sinned, and cursed God in their hearts" (Job 1:5).

Job appears to be the ultimate model of humanity, easily recognized today as the successful, church-going woman or man
who has achieved the American dream of personal and material wealth. Both Job and today's successful people give every
appearance of being invulnerable.

In the first exchange between God and Satan, Poet Job continues to establish that Job's good and upright behavior is not
contingent upon God's continued blessing of his life. The story
tells how Job experiences the loss of everything material which
gave meaning to his life. The Sabeans killed his servants and
stole his oxen and donkeys; the fire of God burned his sheep
and consumed more servants.

Job's troubles continue when the Chaldeans carried off his
camels while killing other servants. His children were killed

when a great wind collapsed their house. No matter how devastated he was by these losses, "Job did not sin or charge God with wrongdoing" (Job 1:22). As if all this were not enough, God allows Satan to inflict "loathsome sores on Job from the sole of his foot to the crown of his head" (Job 2:7).

At the end of the prologue, Job sits silently, totally vulnerable, in the depth of loss. In the presence of his friends, Eliphaz the Temanite, Bildad the Shuhite and Zophar the Naamathite, Job begins his journey through grief. During this process he throws off the cloak of pragmatic religious practice and self-centered endeavors to not only critique, deepen and transform his traditional beliefs but to acknowledge his human vulnerability. In this vulnerability God enters into Job's humanity to become a viable part of Job's world-picture.

The poetic dialogue sections (Job 3:1–42:6) reveal the processing of Job's pain and suffering in the community of his friends. Alteration of his self-image occurs. He struggles to incorporate his past life, present loss and a theocentric cosmology into a new world-picture.

Job's self-alteration destroys the anthropological focused world-picture to reveal an interrelated universe in which God's active voice "calls people to life,"[53] action and witness. This inbreaking of God, this theophany, shatters Job's self-centered ego, concerned only about material loss. Job is then free to engage the mystery and wonder of the cosmos.

The presence of God is manifested to Job and becomes a part of his new world-picture. Job's awareness of God is real and unique to him. It becomes his epiphany. This manifestation of God occurs for Job in a covenantal convergence as his self-identity alters to accept his human vulnerability, his pain, his suffering and his new image of God. Job recognizes his inability to have answers for everything but also recognizes that the God of the theophany is the same God of his religious tradition:

> I had heard of you by the hearing of the ear,
>    but now my eye sees you (Job 42:5).

## Vulnerability

In our present world-pictures, pragmatic religious traditions frequently give a false sense of security, in denial of our real vulnerability. To be human, however, is to be vulnerable. Every child, woman and man has a window of vulnerability in which the inevitability of life's losses will occur. We try to close the windows, cover them up or restrict access to them, but these windows of vulnerability will always be present as long as we live on this earth.

The term "window of vulnerability" is used extensively when military strategists speak about gaps in the defense system which need to be closed.[54] It is an appropriate term to use in a time of AIDS because terminology for disease frequently references the military language of enemy, invader, battle, war and defense.[55] Clinicians also use the word "vulnerability" when discussing opportunistic disease, T-cell status and viral-load in HIV+ patients. These and others are constant reminders of our vulnerability and the massive openings for pain and suffering to enter into our lives.

Job experienced his window of vulnerability. Likewise, countless people today recognize their own windows of vulnerability in the HIV pandemic. Nonetheless, human beings do everything in their power to be safe, to erect safeguards, to keep things the same, to resist change and to be as minimally vulnerable as possible. Job, you and I do not want to admit to being vulnerable.

In his efforts to be invulnerable, Job performed his sacrificial duties scrupulously. Many of us attend church every Sunday because we feel we should rather than because we want to. Dorothee Soelle, however, argues that a window of vulnerability is an essential part of human existence and that it has to stay open for precisely that reason.[56]

Windows let in light, allow us to see out and to be seen. Windows, therefore, expose us and make us vulnerable. Windows represent relationship, receptivity, trust and communication. The human window of vulnerability is also "a window toward heaven"[57] through which epiphany occurs. Unfortunately, when the human experience of pain and suffering washes into our lives it can prompt us to close the windows. Then all becomes darkness and chaos.

### Integrity

If we are willing, Job can teach us how to reopen our windows and how to live in a place of openness and vulnerability. In the beginning of *Job* we meet a man who is presented to us as perfect, a man "blameless and upright, one who feared God and turned away from evil" (Job 1:1). Job was a man who paid attention to the cultic rites of his tradition.

Job was a man who even after losing everything, including his ten children, was able to say:

> Naked I came from my mother's womb, and naked shall I return there; the LORD gave, and the LORD has taken away; blessed be the name of the LORD (Job 1:21).

Job would not "Curse God, and die" (Job 2:9), as his wife suggested.

There can be no question that Job was an exceptional man. God's confidence was justified when God wagered with Satan over disinterested piety during the chilling dialogues of the heavenly court. Job appears to reconcile his loss in the pious expressions of his faith tradition. Job, therefore, was truly the blameless man, the model of integrity. At this point in the story, Job represents the ideal religious response to life's pain and suffering.

The importance of Job's integrity and blameless nature is central to *Job*; the Hebrew word for integrity, *tummah*, is used frequently. However, many commentators argue for this characteristic from the first verse of *Job*:

> There was once a man in the land of Uz whose name was Job. That man was *blameless and upright,* one who feared God and turned away from evil (Job 1:1).

They place great significance upon Poet Job's use of the adjective *tam* to describe Job in the first words of the book, *wehayah ha'ish hahu' tam* (Job 1:1b) to establish Job's integrity and piety.

Janzen describes Job's exemplary response to tragedy by the use of two phrases which establish Job as a man of integrity from the beginning of the story. The first phrase revolves around *tam*, blameless or whole, and *yasar*, upright. This phrase is then juxtaposed with Job's fear of God and turning from evil.

Based on the sentence structure, Janzen argues that Job's uprightness parallels his turning from evil. Job's blamelessness, therefore, parallels his fearing God. Job's blamelessness, consequently, refers to his piety. Job's stoic behavior in the face of tragedy stems from a piety which is genuine and whole. Job's integrity as a man is established.[58]

As mentioned above, Poet Job frequently uses *tummah* to describe Job's integrity. The adjective *tam*, however, is used only twice in the Hebrew Bible (the other time is in Genesis 25:27). Ellen Davis argues that Poet Job's use of *tam* connects Job to another historical figure of integrity. She states:

> the indispensable significance of the word *tam* for understanding Job's character derives from its association with another person of integrity—namely with Jacob—who likewise struggles with God and with Humans (Gen 32:29)—and at last is granted a vision whereby he is fully transformed into the effective vehicle of divine blessing.[59]

The linking of Job's integrity to Jacob is, however, problematic because Jacob is not a blameless man in his early years. Jacob did, after all, steal the birthright of his older brother, Esau (Gen 25:27-34). And it is in the context of these early years that *tam* is used:

> Esau was a skillful hunter, a man of the field while Jacob was as a quiet (*tam*) man, living in tents (Gen 25:27).

and not in his later years as quoted by Davis.

The correct use of *tam* in Job, therefore, refers to a description of Jacob's early life-style. Jacob was the quiet man. He was a person more concerned about being safe, less vulnerable than his brother, Esau, who lived in the vulnerable place of the hunter. Jacob had already begun to build barriers between himself and the natural world. He was a man trying to control his environment.

In assessing the two men's contrasting life-styles, therefore, it can be argued that human social development toward enclosure, social independence, manipulation for material gain and control of the environment was starting to take place in the life-style of Jacob. Jacob, as an archetype of humanity, was beginning to seek ways to lessen humanity's vulnerability. It would, therefore, be appropriate to argue that Poet Job's use of the word *tam* challenges this need to be secure.

In his time, Jacob chose to live in a tent. Now, at the close of the twentieth century, women, children and men live in apartment buildings where neighbor is isolated from neighbor. Material wealth and social position count more than human compassion. The windows of vulnerability seem to be shuttered all around us, as each of us tries to reduce our window of vulnerability to the narrowest slit. And, sadly, this then becomes a place where humanity is most valetudinarian and, therefore, fallible and liable to extremes of pain and suffering.

### Disease/Dis-ease

Humanity is chronically sick, yet wants to be well. In a little known work, *The Meaning of Health*, Paul Tillich states that health can only be known in its relationship to disease: "health is a meaningful term only in confrontation with its opposite—disease."[60] Today, the term "dis-ease" is used more frequently for Tillich's term disease. Dis-ease indicates a feeling of discomfort and/or an ethos of a world-picture not quite right.

Tillich states that the life process includes two basic elements, self-identity and self-alteration. Life takes place in contrasting movement between these elements and is a normal, ongoing process. He explains that the dialectic of this life process can be interrupted by three main causes: accident, intrusion and imbalance. Unfortunately, these causes are rooted in the very ambiguity of the life process. They are, therefore, unavoidable and will cause disease/dis-ease. As Tillich succinctly explains:

> Disease is a symptom of the universal ambiguity of life. Life must risk itself in order to win itself, but in the risking it may lose itself. A life which does not risk disease—even in the highest forms of life of the spirit—is a poor life.[61]

Living is not a stationary process nor is it secure or dependable, however much we try to make it so. The only fixed points of life are birth and death. In between is ambiguity. To live is to risk to be and to change. Therefore, whether we recognize it or not, we constantly encounter elements of transition and change where ambiguity reigns and dis-ease is experienced.

Ambiguity exists because in every creative process of life there is a destructive trend; something is lost and the new is not known. In every integrating process there is a disintegrating; the old world-picture is in transition as it incorporates the new. In every process toward the sublime, a profanizing trend exists; models of the mundane or worldly are used for the ultimate.

The unexpected, the unwanted and the unknown force their way into human awareness to bring trouble and tragedy. These unpredictable events of life also interject trauma into the constant movement between self-identity and self-alteration. Ambiguity is experienced and dis-ease felt as movement takes place.

The dis-ease caused by imbalance can occur because the contrast between self-identity and self-alteration is a dangerous place. There is the danger of losing oneself in either polarity; to be lost when one moves too far beyond the self or to be afraid of losing too much of one's old identity.

Life is not static or stable. Consequently, life always involves ambiguity and the dangerous place between self-identity and self-alteration where dis-ease occurs. Dis-ease, therefore, is at the very center of the life process. This place where disease is felt is where humanity experiences suffering.

## Suffering

A narrow definition of suffering indicates a privation of something good or a change for the worse. This meaning of suffering is the generally accepted one in our society today. However, a broader definition of suffering means undergoing a change either for better or for worse. All life involves constant movement between self-identity and self-alteration; we observe this movement in the daily cycles of night and day, in the birth and death of all living things. In life, change and loss are always present. Therefore, we suffer.

In reality, suffering occurs with change because loss is always present within any change. Each person who risks living will experience the ambiguities and changes of life, and will therefore suffer. We will experience loss and suffering as part of the movement between self-identity and self-alteration. It is up to us to choose to live in the world of opportunity and windows of vulnerability where the risk to change takes place.

Human beings experience change constantly and, therefore, suffer loss even when good things happen. For example, life is drastically changed for a newly married couple with the birth of their first child. Self-identities change; freedom, autonomy and privacy are gone. Although few would express feelings of pain and suffering over these losses,[62] the pain of these changes may frequently linger to later disrupt family relationships.

In a time of AIDS, the magnitude of suffering can be overwhelming as self-identity is constantly being shattered and required to change. The constant change and loss requires unending self-alteration. The ambiguities are enormous and we are challenged to risk greatly if we are to absorb the changes

into our self-identity. The pain of suffering, therefore, is very
great.

## Pain

Pain has its roots in biology and the body's neurological response to felt pain. The neurological response includes reason-
ing, feeling, emotions, memory and changed meaning. Pain is
probably a universal tool for survival by all higher animals.[63]
The human response to pain contains an element of learned
behavior but is also more complex because of the recognized
real and potential change any noxious insult will bring about in
a person's unique life experience.

A noxious insult is something which is injurious or harmful
to health: for example, Job's sores. The pain of such insult does
not necessarily have to have a bodily locus. It may, for example,
affect a person's morale, as Job's life was impacted by the loss
of livelihood and children. A noxious insult will, consequently,
negatively affect the essential and characteristic life process,
activities and functions of a person.

Pain is the initial response of the body to an insult which is
perceived neurologically and/or emotionally by the person.
Change always takes place when pain occurs. The change may
be minimal: a quick stumble on a step causes pain to a big toe
and shakes the person's composure for a minute or two. But it
may also be life shattering, as observed in *Job* where a whole
new identity of personhood and self-identity was forced to
evolve in response to the severity of the losses, the pain, the
fear, and the isolation.

## Pain and Suffering

Women, children and men who experience the physiological pain of AIDS frequently report suffering from pain, rather
than having pain when they feel out of control or at a disad-
vantage. They suffer when a physiological pain is chronic and

overwhelming and dis-ease is felt. Suffering occurs when the source of physiological pain is frequently unknown or the meaning of the pain is a threat to existence.

The core of pain and suffering is an anguish over change which is caused by an injury or a threat of injury and results in the demand to alter the image of self. In the dialectic of life in a global village, demands for change in self-identity are great. Imbalance occurs and the world-picture becomes unstable. Women and men are forced to change. The experience of pain and suffering is great.

### Pain and Suffering in Community

Pain and suffering occur within the human framework of personhood, the multiple conditions of life, character, social structure, cultural background, past history, hopes and expectations, beliefs, understanding of life's meaning, and the obligations of life's roles. Thus, pain and suffering are embedded in the whole human experience, which is sentient and reflective.

Pain and suffering occur when a person's meaning of life is threatened. Pain and suffering will always be experienced and expressed uniquely, according to its historical context. Job experienced and expressed his pain and suffering within the context of his world-picture more than two thousand years ago. I express my pain and suffering within the ethos of my world-picture which has been shaped by my life experiences formed within twentieth-century Western culture.

Pain and suffering do not take place in a vacuum but in the real living of people with each other; thus, they are frequently defined by the community in which they occur. The importance of recognizing how people in community respond to the other's pain and suffering is crucial. For example, a person who experiences pain and suffering under circumstances of relative isolation is often not as verbal when surrounded by a caring and supportive community.

Job's brotherly friends come and sit with him and interact with him as he processes his loss. In the company of Eliphaz the Temanite, Bildad the Shuhite and Zophar the Naamathite Job reflects upon his misery and questions whether or not his pain and suffering is justified. His friends espouse the harsh theology of their tradition, and Job exclaims:

> My companions are treacherous like a torrent-bed,
>     like freshets that pass away,
> that run dark with ice,
>     turbid with melting snow (Job 6:15-16).

A traditional understanding of *hesed* reflects an interdependence of the divine and human dimensions of covenant relationship in which there is an innate fear of God. Norman Habel, on the other hand, prefers the word "brothers" for "companions" or friends and argues that Job needs *hesed* ("loyalty") in his time of crisis:

> In Job's radical understanding of *hesed*, however, human "loyalty" is not necessarily the reflex of divine "loyalty." True "loyalty" is expected from a friend when all other support systems fail, including faith in God.[64]

The companionship of brothers is not a fickle friendship which Job likens to a Palestinian wadi which overflows with water in the rainy season but vanishes when needed (Job 6:15). Poet Job, therefore, presents a radical interpretation of *hesed* that requires "a genuine human compassion and loyalty when all else fails."[65]

It can be argued that Job's brothers have already shown this form of loyalty by sitting with him in silence for seven days among the ashes on a dung heap. They have joined him as an outcast of their society. After Job breaks the silence his friends' courage to continue to be loyal is severely tested by Job's outburst of anger, curse and lament. The language of the texts is bilaterally abusive between Job and the three friends yet communication continues throughout the story.

Even though Job continues to be verbally abusive to his "brothers," they stick by him. They do not get up and walk away. Admittedly, they stay in discourse and conversation to argue their own world-picture. But this debate becomes the sounding board for Job's theological reflections and spiritual growth. How difficult it is to sit with a person as his or her personhood is eroded by AIDS dementia or to stay in friendship as a sister experiences the pain and suffering of end-stage AIDS.

## Stages of Suffering

The pain and suffering of our world is expressed in the anguish of mute suffering, the strident lamentation of transition put into language and the process of change which takes place as the loss is integrated into life.[66] Frequently, suffering is perceived as a change for the worse and reveals the human response to the loss of those things which, today, make a world-picture viable. Today, the universe groans under the weight of the universal suffering caused by AIDS.

Dorothee Soelle, in her book, *Suffering*, describes three phases of suffering.[67] The first phase is a muteness and inability to communicate the anguish of experiencing or observing a threat to the meaning of self. A person is reduced to silence, "they sat with him on the ground . . . and no one spoke a word to him" (Job 2:13). No discourse is possible. Hope is abandoned. Death becomes the only answer. The ability to communicate is almost lost. In the isolation of deep suffering the sufferer turns in upon herself or himself.

If, however, a compassionate friend is willing to sit in the depth of this silence, as Job's three brotherly friends did, then he or she will establish identification and solidarity with the sufferer. The sufferer can then move into the second phase of suffering, expressive suffering. In this phase the expressive compassion of presence—not doing anything but simply being present—allows the sufferer to find language for the pain.

During this second, expressive stage of suffering conversation and dialogue are established through lament, story of past, present and future which must contain elements of truth-telling and honesty. The compassionate friend helps the sufferer name the pain and express through language the grief of loss. The person then moves through rationalization and intellectualization of cultural expectations about loss and grief to, hopefully, experience an epiphany.

Finally, a person moves into the third stage of suffering which creates an acceptable world-picture which gives life meaning and incorporates both the experience of suffering, a life which has value and, hopefully, the presence of God. The three stages of suffering continue to occur throughout the life process as women and men risk self-identity and self-alteration within windows of vulnerability.

A reader of *Job* will recognize her or his own emotions of suffering in a time of AIDS, as the poetic author of this ancient book reveals the human responses to suffering. The first stage, muteness, is personified in the brothers' silent companionship. The second, expressive stage is proclaimed when Job says:

> I will speak in the anguish of my spirit;
> I will complain in the bitterness of my soul (Job 7:11).

The language of pain and suffering continues throughout the dialogue cycles only to end after God has appeared to Job from the whirlwind in the prologue. The reader becomes aware that Job's life goes on where loss has occurred. The changes which tragedy had brought are now incorporated into his ever changing world-picture. He has successfully moved into the third stage of suffering.

## Stages of Loss

The five stages of dying identified by Elisabeth Kubler-Ross may be applied to any loss. Each of these stages—denial/isolation, anger, bargaining, depression and acceptance[68]—is recognizable in Job's story and exemplified in many of Job's utterances. Today, we hear of similar loss in the stories and expressions of persons affected by the HIV/AIDS pandemic.

Kubler-Ross's stages of dying/loss are not meant to describe clearly defined stages but rather the range of human emotions weaving in and out of the human experience of loss and suffering. Denial may be transient or extended. Denial can represent perceived or literal isolation from society. It is important to remember that you can not deny something you do not know! Bargaining is rarely as blatant as Job's, and depression is often harder to detect. Anger, however, remains the dominant and, if directed correctly, healthy emotion.

Acceptance for the sufferer during the HIV pandemic may not be death but life with new meaning. Job was required to let go of his individualism and to accept his lack of power in the frightening and fascinating world of ecological interdependence, relationship and encounter:

> Then the LORD answered Job out of the whirlwind: . . .
> "Look at Behemoth,
>     which I made just as I made you; . . .
> It is the first of the great acts of God—
>     only its Maker can approach it with the sword.
> For the mountains yield food for it
>     where all the wild animals play . . .
> The lotus trees cover it for shade;
>     the willows of the wadi surround it"
>         (Job 40:6, 15, 19–20, 22).

Job's destitute position, his window of vulnerability, became a chasm. But into this chasm broke the opportunity to process the suffering triggered by loss; and, in the end, a covenantal convergence occurs. Poet Job reveals how the power of human imagination and relationship can awaken the soul. He shows how humanity can experience God in the midst of pain and suffering.

# Reflection

At the start of my night shift I walked into the room of a new patient who had been admitted that afternoon with a diagnosis of End Stage AIDS. From the medical report I knew that while hospitalized she had had an adverse medication reaction which had affected her limbs. Now she was close to death. Nothing could have prepared me for what I saw. The isolation of the hospital bed in the center of the room, not touching wall, table or window, was explained as "a precautionary measure; she hits out at everything." As I moved closer the frail shadow of a twenty-one-year-old human being appeared no more than a waif of a woman. Her face was averted from me, no voice responded to my "Hello" and introduction. Her eyelids fluttered over closed eyes. Silence prevailed, permeating the space between us.

Later, angry grunts and groans greeted the evening routine of nursing care. Her hands and feet had been turned to cold, stone-like blackened claws by medications meant to help her. She lay, this young mother, dependent on our care, ostracized by her family and isolated by her pain and suffering. Food was refused by a mouth clamped shut, light was denied through lids held tightly closed and touch was limited to the intravenous line for pain medication and artificial nutrition.

Day by day, night by night we cared for her as best we could. It became my custom to sit in her room and do my charting at the end of my shift. No words were spoken between us. One evening when I came into her room at the start of my shift I noticed the eyelids flutter and open for a brief second. Nothing more.

Then one night, after I had been gone for a few days, as I settled in the chair by her bed to do my nightly charting I heard the richest words in the world, "Where you been?" "Oh, off for a few days." Nothing more was ever said between us, but the groans and grunts lessened as we turned and changed her. Soon life slipped out of her frail, waif-like form.

The mist and rain hid the sunlight as my car climbed the winding road of the canyon as I drove home. "Why?" I asked the silent, bowed and burdened rain-laden trees beside me. "She was so young," I complained to the crystal drops of rain glistening in my headlights. "God, it's not fair," I cried, as I groped my way around the last bends of the familiar road.

Suddenly, sunlight flooded my path as I reached the top of the canyon. My way was now clear but the mist wrapped its cold fingers through the clefts in the hills below me. I watched a hawk fly high in the air currents as she looked for prey to feed her young ones. Suddenly, she swooped to grasp the living food in her lethal, cold claws.

I felt the universe's pain and suffering.

---

An outpouring of pain and suffering was innate to the catastrophic loss Job experienced and we experience in a time of AIDS.

However much we would like to minimize our window of vulnerability we are unable to do so.

The pain and suffering associated with the AIDS pandemic is monumental and universal.

Many people with AIDS were, and still are, pushed to the "dung heap" of society. Those who stay with them are also designated as belonging there.

Today we experience the overwhelming silence when words are inadequate to express our pain and suffering in a time of AIDS.

How hard it is for us to sit in silence for even a few minutes with a friend who is dying.

We are often drowned by a deluge of words as an outpouring of this pain sweeps over us.

We also recognize that lives continue all around us with the pain and suffering incorporated into joyful living.

The knowledge of individual and cumulative loss is so great.

Loss has to be processed so that life can go on. The processing of loss is multifaceted but occurs when a person can be in a community which understands and affirms her or his pain and suffering.

*Job* reveals to me a praxis for processing the pain and suffering associated with loss.

*Job* requires me to give up my need for control and to acknowledge that as a human being I am vulnerable and constantly involved in change.

*Job* challenges me to accept this vulnerability so that I can experience the in-breaking of God into a world devastated by the HIV virus and AIDS.

*Job* is a message of hope and help I need in a time of AIDS. It has taught me to accept my human vulnerability. Epiphany has occurred for me in the glint of sunlight, rain-burdened bows, rivers of moss, people taking care of each other, circles of prayer and in community.

# – 6 –

# Job Speaks

Then Job answered:
  "O that my vexation were weighed,
  and all my calamity laid in the balances!
For then it would be heavier than the sand of the sea; . . ."
  (Job 6:1-3).

Today, we live in community with each other in a global village where the pain of the "other" is, and must be, "ours." For
humanity has AIDS. The lament and curse text, Job 3:1-26, is
an example of a biblical text which reveals the human experiential response of anger to the pain and suffering innate to the
HIV pandemic.

Job's first lament and curse passage, which breaks the seven-
day silence, affirms that anger, rage and bitterness are very
human feelings. These are neither evil nor sinful feelings; and
there is a need for an honest admission that "anger is simply
one of the subjects the faithful take to God."[69]

For seven days Job and his brotherly friends sit in silence
(Job 2:13). The world is without language and has, therefore,
returned to primordial chaos. Job's life is without meaning,
form or future. This same type of chaos has entered our universe
in a time of AIDS. Job, when he starts to curse and lament,
does not know what his future will be. He does not know he
will see God. The anguish just explodes. As Job moves out of

the silent stage of his affliction, a change in his self-identity starts to take place.

At this point there is, of course, a risk. The risk of vulnerability and of letting go. A willingness to change and to trust in God is necessary, and commitment not to bring revenge upon another is essential. Nonetheless, feelings as dreadful as Job's death wish, shocking as they are, need to be vocalized. Job leads the way.

**Imprecation**

Job's imprecation starts with seven curses followed by lament (Job 3:1-26). In acute despair Poet Job's powerful words bring multiple images of the darkness of the primordial chaos which existed before life was formed. Job starts by cursing the day of his birth:

> Let that day be darkness!
>> May the God above not seek it,
>> or light shine on it.
> Let gloom and deep darkness claim it (Job 3:4-5).

Poet Job constantly contrasts light with darkness, day to night, life and death, birth to death, order against chaos, knowledge with mystery throughout this passage. These words are reminders of the immeasurable dichotomies which fill human existence.

In the idiomatic, dramatic language of the Semite, who is not ashamed to curse and bless, Job's rage bursts forth. He dares to curse[70] not only the day of his birth, but even the time of his pre-birth, the night of his conception:

> and the night that said,
> 'a man-child is conceived' (Job 3:3b).

The multiple incantations which follow Job's initial outburst express his physical and spiritual misery. Through powerful cosmological mythic images, they summon forth darkness, barrenness, oblivion and chaos:

> Yes, let that night be barren;
> let no joyful cry be heard in it.
> Let those curse it who curse the Sea,
> those who are skilled to rouse up Leviathan.
> Let the stars of its dawn be dark;
> let it hope for light, but have none; (Job 3:7-9).

These are the powers necessary to obliterate God's gift of created being, life.

The seven incantations about the day of his birth (Job 3:11-26) assault creation and destroy the structure of temporal order. Fertility and procreation turn to sterility. Job wishes to escape into the nothingness of death.

God, Job believes, has humanity hedged in as the waters were controlled at creation (Job 38:8) not for protection, as Satan's comments would have us believe (Job 1:10), but to obfuscate the light necessary for humanity to find its way (Job 3:23). In this time of AIDS the creation feels stifled, strangled and suffocated as the HIV stealthily encroaches upon the very breath of human life.

Job even risks reversal of creation when he offers the challenge to call upon "those who are skilled to rouse up Leviathan" (Job 3:8). Leviathan can return the world to pre-creation darkness. Job believes that only in gloom and darkness can the evil day of his birth be redeemed.[71] Then it will be obscured from memory. Nothing, it appears, is worth living for. He has no fear, nothing to lose in the torment of his spirit. At this time he exists without hope or knowledge of God. He can damn himself into oblivion.

The theme of the initial outburst of curse, lament and death-wish, becomes more subdued and bitter as Job continues in classic lament form. All the hurt, pain, dis-ease and dissonance of Job's life are evoked by his language in this passage; the language justifies the term "lament" even if the traditional sequences are not overtly observed.[72] Job cries:

> Why did I not die at birth,
> come forth from the womb and expire?
> Why were there knees to receive me,
> or breasts for me to suck? (Job 3:11-12)

Job's petition is to die and go where "the wicked cease from troubling, and there the weary rest" (Job 3:17). His lament extends beyond a self-lament to incorporate all people who live lives of misery:

> Why is light given to one in misery,
> and life to the bitter in soul,
> who long for death, but it does not come (Job 3:20-21).

Job longs for death, to be out of his misery, just as a woman recently diagnosed with AIDS longs for release from the torment of psoriasis. Job's bold, risky and shocking language finally confronts the hard existential reality of a life of sickness devoid of children, home and livelihood. A woman lying isolated in a hospital bed, shunned by her friends, visited reluctantly by her family and dependent upon Medi-Cal for medical treatment will instantly recognize the hard existential reality of isolation.

Both Job and this woman have lost the relationships and things which have value for them and have given meaning to their lives. Life itself no longer has meaning and they are totally vulnerable. Job believes his enemy is his life and, therefore, the one who gave him life, God. Many people experiencing AIDS feel this way and some courageously verbalize these feelings.

Job's enemy is the same God whom Satan challenged as Job's protector at the beginning of the story:

> Does Job fear God for nothing? Have you not put a fence around him and his house and all that he has, on every side? (Job 1:9-10)

The enemy for Job, justifiably, appears in the text as the very God who has allowed Job's material, physical and emotional world to be destroyed. This is a world recognized today as filled with rage evoking pain, sickness, loss and grief. They remove the meaning from life and appear to proliferate without restraint in a time of AIDS.

Poet Job concludes Job's first soliloquy on his suffering by referencing that the hedges God created about him for sustenance and protection, as mentioned above, have now become the bonds which bind him to a life of pain bereft of light. The final three verses have tremendous rhetorical power as they integrate a number of related terms:

> For my sighing comes like my bread,
>  and my groanings are poured out like water.
> Truly the thing that I fear comes upon me,
>  and what I dread befalls me (Job 3:24-25).

The final verse is a catalytic summary of Job's lament:

> I am not at ease, nor am I quiet;
> I have no rest; but trouble comes (Job 3:26).

In these final words of Job's first speech there is a repetition of the motif of trouble and turmoil[73] combined with the restless verb "to come." Poet Job knows trouble and turmoil are an integral and upsetting part of human existence. These words set a tone of restlessness for the following dialogue cycles.

There is no peace or rest or quiet for those who suffer in a time of AIDS. There is only turmoil, dissonance, disorder, chaos, pain and suffering for women, children, and men infected or affected by the HIV virus. But Job has dared to speak aloud the concealed and terrible anguish of the suffering human spirit and response is demanded.

Job is not alone. His brotherly friends from afar, Eliphaz the Temanite, Bildad the Shuhite and Zophar the Naamathite are with him and enter into conversation with him. Job now begins a verbal journey out of affliction into the anger of expressive suffering. The darkness of despair and lament turns to anger and revolt as Job responds to the three friends' orthodox religious arguments for unexplainable human suffering.

## Conversation: Eliphaz

"If one ventures a word with you, will you be offended?" (Job 4:2) are the tentative words Eliphaz the Temanite uses to start conversation with Job. Eliphaz begins by affirming Job's life and speaks of him as a man who has advised others in time of trouble. Eliphaz then proceeds to expound upon a reality which acknowledges that humans are not pure, "are born to trouble" (Job 5:7) and God metes out justice. Job is no different and must, therefore, have sinned because he is now suffering. Eliphaz argues Job's only hope is to repent and turn to God who will redeem him.

## Job Reflects on Eliphaz's Speech

Job's first responses to Eliphaz's verbalization of this classic, retribution-based theodicy, is to acknowledge the effect of this theology on the human psyche. Using all the power of metaphorical language, Poet Job speaks for humanity's suffering soul when Job cries:

> For the arrows of the Almighty are in me;
> my spirit drinks their poison (Job 6:4).

Job continues to reflect upon his misery in the death-wish of lament, wallowing in self-pity (6:2-3a). He then starts to question whether the pain and suffering are justified (6:8-30). Job continues not only to challenge the truth of what Eliphaz has said but also to turn upon his friend to question the kindness of a constant espousal of the harsh doctrine of retribution (Job 6:14-17). In this passage Job becomes a raucous reminder for us not to preach retribution theology in a time of AIDS.

Job ends his first speech not to plead for divine deliverance but to speak of his trust in God. Now Job begins to dialogue with the established theology of retribution as he moves into active complaint, protest and accusations:

> Therefore I will not restrain my mouth;
>> I will speak in the anguish of my spirit;
>> I will complain in the bitterness of my soul.
> Am I the Sea, or the Dragon,
>> that you set a guard over me? (Job 7:11-12).

## Job on the Human Condition

Job begins to reflect back to his lamentation and to discern how God's past relationship with him fits into the present situation. Job recognizes the universal hardship and slavery of the human condition. Job falls into an introspection upon his life and the realization that, within traditional Israelite theology, existence is perceived to be hard service to a super-taskmaster, a "watcher of humanity" (Job 7:20). Job's soul-searching about human existence contrasts sharply with Eliphaz's quick and easy rote answer for the causation of trouble to be sin.

Poet Job's reflections on the human condition (Job 7:1-21) identify three axioms of human existence: servitude, futility and humiliation. In commenting on the first axiom of servitude, Habel remarks that Poet Job had an awareness of the Near Eastern myths which saw humans as created specifically for the purpose of liberating deities from mundane tasks.[74]

Habel and Janzen both indicate that the Hebrew word *saba'* tends to be used (480 times) in relationship to military service (1 Kgs 9:15-22; cf. 2 Chr 26:11) and only in Isaiah 40:2, "She (Jerusalem) has served her term" and in *Job* is the context "slave service" used:

> Do not human beings have a hard service on earth,
>> and are not their days like the days of laborer?
> Like a slave who longs for the shadow (Job 7:1-2).

Nonetheless, Poet Job chooses this word deliberately either in remembrance of Israel's time of exile or, perhaps, to emphasize religious servitude.[75] Job is obviously feeling very miserable, enslaved, and burdened by his life.

The second axiom, futility of life, focuses on the irreversibility of mortality:

> My days are swifter than a weaver's shuttle,
>     and come to their end without hope (Job 7:6).

Poet Job tells us life is transitional. We are all born with the terminal condition: death. Poet Job, at this point, does not deny humanity's mortality. He endeavors, by using the metaphorical symbols of chaos, to alert God to the enormity of the human crisis[76] when pain, suffering and death enter life. Job then exemplifies the discomfort and dis-ease of living with AIDS:

> When I say 'My bed will comfort me,
>     my couch will ease my complaint,'
> then you scare me with dreams
>     and terrify me with visions,
> so that I would choose strangling
>     and death rather than this body.
> I loathe my life; I would not live forever.
>     Let me alone, for my days are a breath (Job 7:13-16).

The final axiom is to reveal how pain and suffering bring humility into human existence. Job now speaks words of irony, wordplay and double entendres to bring home the humble reality of human existence. The poet's specific choice of words, all with double meanings—"shade/shadow" (7:2), "thread/hope" (7:7), "spirit/wind" (7:9), and "throat/life" (7:15)—project the depth of Job's anguish and Poet Job's understanding of humanity's humble, painful lot in life.[77]

Finally, Poet Job parodies Psalm 8 which affirms the Israelite tradition of a caring God who created women and men in the image of God. The psalmist, in Psalm 8, speaks of an awesome sense of majesty within the cosmos and a subsequent realization of the majesty of the creator in contrast to human mortality and fallibility.

Nonetheless, the psalmist indicates this frail human is called into a higher vocation with the creator:

> What are human beings that you are mindful of them,
>> mortals that you care for them?
> Yet you have made them a little lower than God
>> (Psalm 8:4-5).

The psalmist believed humanity to be the exalted servants who have dominion over the works of God's hands. But this image is de-constructed as Job claims humanity is God's prey instead of God's regent:

> What are human beings, that you make so much of them,
>> that you set your mind on them,
> visit them every morning,
>> test them every moment?
> Will you not look away from me for a while,
>> let me alone until I swallow my spittle? (Job 7:17-19)

Poet Job has turned Psalm 8 upside down and asks God why mortal humanity is of so much interest to the creator. Poet Job's irony of Psalm 8 makes Job mock God as a plague to humanity, watching, spying and bothering it each day with a new set of tests and troubles. Job denies the image of God and humanity together bringing the light of life to the cosmos each day.

Instead of the joyful and creative union of humanity with God, as envisioned by the psalmist, Job quotes the futility of all human life which ends in dust. Finally, Job ends his first speech taunting God that when God seeks for humanity, made in God's image, it will not exist:

> For now I shall lie in the earth;
>> for you will seek me, but I shall not be (Job 7:21).

The in-depth use of irony for the parody of Psalm 8 becomes crucial for the rest of the book because it creates the cradle in which Job's growth is nurtured. The deep darkness of silent suffering has been released. Job now begins the process of seeking a God who will eventually appear to him in the whirlwind to turn his world around.

## Conversation: Bildad

The second friend, Bildad the Shuhite, enters into the discourse. He is much more blunt than Eliphaz. He comes straight to the point. God would not make a mistake by perverting justice. Bildad rhetorically presents the pragmatic rationale for pain and suffering:

> If your children sinned against him,
>> he delivered them into the power of their transgression
>> (Job 8:4).

Poet Job knew, just as we do, that the laws of cause and effect apply to human existence. Women and men, therefore, must take responsibility for acts which bring pain and suffering, sickness and death. AIDS is a preventable syndrome because we know it is caused by the HIV retrovirus transmitted primarily through blood and genital fluids.

Stopping the HIV pandemic is possible and prevention must be taught from an intellectual perspective. But responding to the pain and suffering the disease causes requires not only this intellectual response but an encapsulation of the pragmatic within a compassionate ethos of caring which does not pass judgment.

## Job's Response to Bildad's Speech

Job begins his response to Bildad by demanding, "How can a man be just before God?" (Job 9:2) when God has all the power. God, Job believes, is using his power to destroy Job, "for he crushes me with a tempest" (Job 9:17). The God who defeated chaos to make the creation has now turned against the creation.

God, Job argues, appears to destroy both the blameless and the wicked. God is wicked and corrupt. Job's integrity confronts in terror his passion to prove himself innocent before a God who appears to be powerful, malicious and capricious. Job is willing to risk his life, for his life has lost its value.

## Job on the Relationship between God and Humanity

Job acknowledges the chasm he feels between humanity and God, "for he is not a mortal, as I am" (Job 9:32). Now he starts to probe the reality of God. Job asks innumerable questions in response to Bildad's narrow interpretation for pain and suffering. In this way he reaches out toward God as the measure of all things.

Job has become aware that God has neither the eyes of flesh nor the sense of human time (Job 10:4-5) and place. Yet Job realizes that there is a relationship between God and the creation. Job has accepted his creation by God, God's love for the creation and humanity's mortality:

> Remember that you fashioned me like clay;
>     and will you turn me to dust again? . . .
> You clothed me with skin and flesh,
>     and knit me together with bones and sinews.
> You have granted me life and steadfast love,
>     and your care has preserved my spirit (Job 10:9-12).

Job now understands. God's love and care for humanity is not within the realm of finite material wealth or the physical body. God cares for the human spirit: "your care has preserved my spirit" (Job 10:12). Job, in his refusal to believe the orthodox retribution theology, has found in his reflective questions to God the message that God cannot keep pain and suffering out of human life. Yet God does care for and preserve the human spirit, always.

Poet Job forcefully reminds us that God grants us life, gives us steadfast love and cares for our spirits. Deep in the universality of God's heart exists the awesome compassion that cares for creation regardless of our behavior. This is the heart which holds the quilts of all people who have died from HIV. Job speaks for us when he accuses God that "these things you hid in your heart" (Job 10:13). Sometimes, when we are suffering and deep in depression it is hard to remember God's steadfast love for our souls.

### Conversation: Zophar

Zophar the Naamathite now castigates Job for his garrulous prattling:

> Should a multitude of words go unanswered,
>     and should one full of talk be vindicated?
> Should your babble put others to silence,
>     and when you mock, shall no one shame you? (Job 11:2-3)

Poet Job introduces a trace of the future theophany when he has Zophar articulate the inability of humanity to understand the cosmos:

> Can you find out the deep things of God?
>     Can you find out the limit of the Almighty? (Job 11:7)

Zophar next appears to call Job stupid and slow to understand:

> But a stupid person will get understanding,
>     when a wild ass is born human (Job 11:12).

Zophar's theology says Job is guilty because he is suffering. Zophar piously states that all will be well if Job would only turn to God in humble obedience ("stretch out your hands" [Job 11:13]) and eliminate evil from his life ("do not let wickedness reside in your tents" [Job 11:14]). If Job drops all deceit ("Lift up your face without blemish" [Job 11:15]), his pain and suffering will cease.[78]

## Job Reflects on Zophar's Speech

Job argumentatively responds to Zophar. Wisdom and knowledge belong to God, which observation of the natural world proves:

> But ask the animals, and they will teach you;
> the birds of the air, and they will tell you;
> ask the plants of the earth, and they will teach you;
> and the fish of the sea will declare to you (Job 12:7-8).

> Look, my eye has seen all this,
> my ear has heard and understood it (Job 13:1).

Job will not accept Zophar's remedies of pious behavior which he perceives as hypocrisy. Job ends by accusing Zophar of speaking falsely and deceitfully for God (Job 13:7).

## Job on Retribution Theology

Job has now established for himself a rebuttal to the established Hebrew religious tradition's justification for pain and suffering. He claims Zophar's "maxims are proverbs of ashes," his "defenses are defenses of clay" (Job 13:12). Job girds himself in his integrity, innocence and vulnerability. Knowing he is mortal he is willing to face his God. He asks two things of God:

> Withdraw your hand from me,
> and do not let dread of you terrify me (Job 13:21).

Job has stated his case and is willing to be in conversation with God.

The first cycle concludes with Job enunciating for all time the finitude and fragility of the human condition. He then exhibits humanity's eternal optimism when he muses upon the possibility of return from Sheol to prove his innocence before a less vengeful God. Job returns to his lament ethos and the cycle ends with Job accusing God of destroying the hope of all mortals.

**The Argument**

The verbal exchanges continue. The friends stay and speak the pious beliefs of their orthodox religion. Job, on the other hand, reaches deep within his soul to express the anguish of his experiences of loss. His life is now burdensome and consists of endless pain and suffering. He is a desperate man. He is deep within the chasm of vulnerability. In this place of vulnerability Job is free to see God.

The dialogue cycles draw to a close and Job appears to argue more with himself and God than in direct response to the brotherly friends' speeches. His angry argument before God is based upon his observation of the cosmological patterns of interrelationship, consistency and repetition in the natural world of creation through which God develops order and structure. Disparity exists: things do not fit.

God, Job indicates, is revealed in the created order of the cosmos but all he, Job, has experienced recently has been destruction of order. His social life is in ruin and his body is racked by sickness. Chaos, not God, appears to reign.

The brotherly friends describe Job as foolish to revolt against and attack God. Job, however, reverses the metaphors and makes it the divine ruler attacking him, a weak, defenseless mortal. Job makes an oath of innocence and revolt (Job 29–31). Alone, he calls upon God to hear him:

> Oh, that I had one to hear me!
>     (Here is my signature! Let the Almighty answer me!)
>     Oh that I had the indictment written by my adversary!
> Surely I would carry it on my shoulder;
>     I would bind it on me like a crown;
> I would give him an account of all my steps;
> like a prince I would approach him (Job 31:35-37).

Job proclaims his integrity for all to hear. He casts off the orthodox theology of retribution and stands tall in the conviction of his innocence as a human being. The challenge has been brought to God: if God keeps silent, then God is guilty of the charges Job brings.

## Breakdown

The third cycle of conversation (Job 22–27) between Job and his brotherly friends does not follow the preceding pattern. The cycle begins as the others do: Eliphaz is answered by Job. But as chapter 24 begins, the reader notes a different speech pattern. The speaker is assumed to be Job but, rather than appealing to God in lament form as he has done previously, he poses questions for debate or dispute. Job begins to sound like his friends.

What is being said, by whom and why? Job starts by asking where is God when he, Job, is experiencing all this pain and suffering? In typical Joban language the reader hears of Job's innocent suffering as at the hands of oppressors: "they drive away the donkey of the orphan; . . . they thrust the needy off the road" (Job 24:3, 4).

Job expresses antiphonally the state of the oppressed to be "Like wild asses in the desert they go out to their toil, . . . lie all night naked, . . . cling to the rock for want of shelter" (Job 24:5, 7, 8). The human plight of poverty, exploitation, hunger, injustice and evil is poignantly represented in multiple symbolic ways. People suffer and there is no retribution from God.

The difficulty begins as the brotherly friends' doctrines of retribution for evildoers are heard "so wickedness is broken like a tree" (Job 24:20). Could Job say these words? It is at this point that many scholars see dislocation in the cycle and suggest alternate ways of compiling this chapter. Some scholars would add this portion of Job's speech to Bildad's third cycle speech or to Zophar's. But the theme of retribution theology does not fit well with either speech. Thus, these scholars hear Bildad, not Job, repeating the familiar theme of God's power and dominion over sinful humanity (Job 24:18-24); and they hear Zophar reiterating his previous speech on the fate of the wicked (Job 27:7-23).[79]

There exists, however, a coherent thesis for this passage if it is seen as a Joban soliloquy. Job is in debate with himself. He is juxtaposing the traditional Hebraic understanding of retribution and his own observations of pain and suffering in the world. In other words, in this speech Poet Job has encapsulated in Job's speech the whole previous dialogue cycles. The traditional teachings of orthodox religions are challenged by Job's experience of loss. Finally, Poet Job puts into the mouth of Job humanity's eternal lament when God seems silent in times of tragedy:

> From the city the dying groan,
> and the throat of the wounded cries for help;
> yet God pays no attention to their prayer (Job 24:12).

Job has explored his pain to the depth of his soul. He has verbalized his suffering in anger and rage at God. After multiple imprecations, outbursts of anger and lament, Job has realized the awesome nature of the creation and accepted the mystery of God's apparent absence.

Job's angry outbursts, reflections and interaction have become the agents of change for himself in his relationship with himself, others and God. His world-picture is being re-created, self-alteration has started to occur.

This process has taken place in the companionship of his brotherly friends who have stuck with him. In the depth of his pain and suffering change has occurred. The anger of the anguished spirit is surrendered but not suppressed and God has the freedom to intervene.

The process of the transitions between self-identity and self-alteration within an ethos of conversation within his faith tradition is changing Job's world-picture. Job is vulnerable and aware of God's steadfast love and care for the human spirit. Job's willingness to be vulnerable enables him to move into his spiritual awakening (epiphany). A space is opened up for the in-breaking of God.

# Reflection

The voice droned on about the rules and regulations for the Hospice Benefit. My mind followed the words as my soul followed the persons suffering from HIV/AIDS waiting for my care. My memory sought those who had died from the pandemic in the past few weeks, days and years. I found myself angry. There was such a void in my heart between the cold facts being spoken and the reality of my emotions.

Intellectually, I know that anger is a part of the processing of my grief, but how to reconcile the sight of a person in their twenties or thirties, skin as taut as a drum spread over bones which stick out, covered with the scales of psoriasis and no longer able to recognize mother or daughter—how to reconcile this terrible sight with the comfortable and composed ethos of nursing education?

Where is the outlet for the frustration of one day being by the bedside of a dying person and the next day having to walk into another home devastated by tragedy? How can a person cope with the knowledge that in a few weeks, or even days, this woman, man or child will be joining her or his cold sisters and brothers in premature graves.

I remember looking down as I left a home after a death and seeing the gentle river of moss between the macadam and the concrete of the road. Surviving even under the constant battering of traffic. I remember feeling like the macadam of the road. I remember being comforted by a letter of thanks from the daughters.

I remember carrying an AIDS quilt banner in procession down a busy campus street to a memorial service. I and the others in procession walked through the crowds as though we were invisible. I remember sitting in silence with the young woman, withered, wasted and wan. I remember hugging the four generations of women and glancing over their shoulders at the Bible on top of the television, open to *Job*.

I am not quiet, nor am I at ease today.

I remember the note given to another nurse struggling to bring light into the world in a time of AIDS. It had a sad face at the top and words of powerlessness, sadness, tiredness, diseases and the plea to be kept out of pain cascading like tears on the white paper. But as the words dried up a metamorphosis had taken place.

In the place of despair, pain and suffering, now were words of gratitude and the banishment of fear. For hope returns in the expressions of caring. Hope comes each morning as the red skirts of dawn push away the darkness of despair.

As it has so often in the past, verbalization of memory has come to heal the soul. I remember that a hundred years ago Soren Kierkegaard identified Job with the angry voice of human pain and had the courage to admit "Thee I have need of, a man who knows how to complain aloud."[80]

The need continues today in a time of AIDS.

————————

Job's imprecation, his outburst of anger, is a good starting place for the expression of human anguish in a time of AIDS.

All people, if they are honest with themselves, will admit that at some tragic or miserable time in their lives they have questioned the meaning of life.

They may even have had the courage to verbalize a death wish; some, tragically, have taken their own lives. Job, therefore, speaks the universal cry of anguish when he breaks the silence of the dung heap.

Job reminds us that anger is an emotion and does not need to be legitimized or justified. It just is and stems from deep emotions of fear, hurt and anxiety.

Poet Job verbalizes, through the mouths of the friends, the Israelite views on causation of pain and suffering as coming from God. Strong traces of this theology exist today.

The verbal exchanges which follow speak of humanity's experiences of pain and suffering and religion's response.

We reflect upon our experiences to critique, deepen and transform our religious traditions in a time of AIDS.

The three axioms identified by Job as innate to human existence remind us that life is hard, humbling and finite.

We are also reminded that we can not escape from the responsibility of our actions.

Job is also that raucous reminder for us not to preach retribution theology in a time of AIDS and to stay faithful with our sisters and brothers in their times of dissonance, disorder, chaos, pain and suffering.

# – 7 –

# Epiphany

Then the LORD answered Job out of the whirlwind:
"Where were you when I laid the foundation of the earth?
   Tell me, if you have understanding.
Who determined its measurements—surely you know!
   Or who stretched the line upon it?
On what were its bases sunk,
   or who laid its cornerstone
when the morning stars sang together
   and all the heavenly beings shouted for joy?"
      (Job 38:1, 4-7).

Job's covenanting convergence takes place in the experience
of God appearing to him in a whirlwind; it is the source of Job's
epiphany, his spiritual awakening. This covenanting convergence
transforms his perspective on the character of God and requires
him to reflect upon his own place and purpose in the world. The
convergence between God and Job reveals the powerful imaginative theology innate to Poet Job's Hebrew world-picture.

In the previous chapters of *Job*, we have witnessed the painful
journey of the man named Job who lived in the land of Uz. We
have heard the story of an innocent man who experienced great
pain and suffering. We have known of a wager between God and
Satan which was unknown to Job and his friends.

Our hearts and souls have been filled with metaphors for
the dissonance, disorder, chaos, pain and suffering which Job

felt two thousand years ago—and which we experience be-cause of the HIV pandemic. The pages have been full of emo-tional storms of loss, pain and grief and Job's temperamental tempest of dissent as he has processed his personal tragedy.

Poet Job, therefore, finds it appropriate to make the theo-phany start with the words: "Then the LORD answered Job out of the whirlwind" (Job 38:1). Not a storm but a whirlwind. Pal-estine is a country of contrast in a small land area which is swept by the searing, devastating forces of the Sirocco wind in Spring and Autumn. This hot, dry wind originates in the Sa-hara and often brings not only temperatures of one hundred and ten degrees with a humidity of two percent but also de-structive storms and tempests.[81]

A great wind had collapsed Job's eldest son's home and all his ten children were dead (Job 1:19). Yahweh, however, does not appear to Job in a storm but in a whirlwind; the de-struction has already occurred and a deluge of emotion has been spent and now God is present to whirl Job around with questions.

Poet Job uses some of the most beautiful language in the Bible in the chapters which speak of God's presence with Job and Job's epiphany. The theophany begins with four strophes (38:4-18)[82] that portray the Hebrew understanding of a cosmos methodically created and ruled by God into four parts: the earth, the sea, the heavens and the underworld. It recalls the order and balance of creation.

The poet speaks of the earth where the morning stars sing together and the heavenly beings shout for joy as the skirts of dawn are shaken:

> On what were its bases sunk,
>     or who laid its cornerstone
> when the morning stars sung together
>     and all the heavenly beings shouted for joy? (Job 38:6-7).

Poet Job's world-picture saw the earth solidly founded on four pillars, covered with the rich garment of God's clouds:

> when I made the clouds its garments,
>> and thick darkness its swaddling band (Job 38:9).

Job believed the earth was lovingly measured and carefully divided by God. God shut the sea with doors and set the boundaries for the waves to keep God's creatures safe from the primordial waters of chaos:

> and (I) prescribed bounds for it,
>> and set bars and doors,
> and said, 'thus far shall you come and no farther,
>> and here shall your proud waves be stopped' (Job 38:10-11).

God even asks Job the ultimate unanswerable question:

> Have the gates of death been revealed to you,
>> or have you seen the gates of deep darkness? (Job 38:17).

In the next six strophes Poet Job uses imaginative creation metaphors of crafting, fertility, word and conflict (38:19-38) to describe the meteorological phenomena of the cosmos. Poet Job uses the familiar words of light and darkness, snow, hail, wind, rain, dew, hoarfrost, ice, the constellations and clouds to paint a picture of a creation constantly being conceived:

> Has the rain a father,
>> or who has begotten the drops of dew?
> From whose womb did the ice come forth,
>> and who has given birth to the hoarfrost of heaven?
>> (Job 38:28-29).

Poet Job has God ask Job if he knows of the heavenly palace above the firmament which contains the storehouses of the snow and hail or "the way to the place where the light is distributed" or where the winds are "scattered upon the earth" (Job 38:24). Poet Job has God speak of the wonder of windows in the dome above the earth. These windows allow the rains to be tipped from waterskins to fall upon the ground regardless of human occupation.

God reminds Job of the constellations which travel their appointed paths upon this dome and the miracle of the presence of light and darkness in the world:

> Where is the way to the dwelling of light,
>     and where is the place of darkness? (Job 38:19).

The metaphor of God as ruler is de-stabilized in the next five strophes (38:39–39:30) and Poet Job ends God's first speech by denying an anthropocentric world. God asks of Job, "Is the wild ox willing to serve you?" (Job 39:9). Poet Job presents the theological paradox of a God who created the cosmos but who is not necessarily in charge but more in relationship with the creation:

> Is it at your command that the eagle mounts up
>     and makes its nest on high?
> It lives on the rock and makes its home
>     in the fastness of the rocky crag.
> From there it spies the prey;
>     its eyes see it from far away.
> Its young ones suck up blood;
>     and where the slain are, there it is (Job 39:27-30).

The zoological groupings of animals and birds by Poet Job are characterized each by a common feature: ravenous appetites, reproduction, freedom, speed and irrational courage, and wisdom. The lion, raven, ibex, wild ass and ox, ostrich and eagle are all wild. They are all recognizable as animals which are perceived to be harmful to human life and non-responsive to domestication. The horse is the only domesticated animal mentioned by Poet Job.[83]

The life and death struggles of the animal world are presented in a harsh, compelling reality where neither the hunted nor the hunter are pitied but exist in a dignity of relationships even when there is perceived to be pain and suffering:

> The ostrich's wings flap wildly,
>     though its pinions lack plumage.

> For it leaves its eggs to the earth,
> > and lets them be warmed on the ground,
> forgetting that a foot may crush them,
> > and that a wild animal may trample them. . . .
> When it spreads its plumes aloft,
> > it laughs at the horse and its rider (Job 39:13-15, 18).

Poet Job proclaims the providential care and feeding of all the animals in creation. The poet has subverted an anthropocentric world-picture. The human need to control for survival is null. The human moral order has no place in the struggle between death and survival for Poet Job.

The lion and raven hunt for prey to feed their young. The mountain goat and calving deer produce their young in their allotted time only to see the young grow strong and leave. The wild ass and ox roam free among the mountaintops and pastures where they disdain all human efforts of control. The speedy ostrich and the majestic war horse laugh at wisdom and at human fears and frailty.

Poet Job observes the hawk soaring high above the earth and the eagle nesting upon a rocky crag. Both the eagle and the hawk will delight to feed on and suck the blood of fallen prey. This is not an anthropocentric world but a world of ecological interdependence, relationship and encounter.

In God's view of creation there is both an "indestructible power and an indestructible joy."[84] God's creation does not exist within the limits of human understanding or the desire to be safe. God can not be contained by legalism or pragmatic piety innate to religious doctrines and dogma. God's creation exists in power, in joy and in free relationships.

God challenges Job to answer but Job's argumentative personality seems to have disappeared. God, therefore, continues and challenges Job either to supplant the mythical gods and do battle with the elements of chaos represented by the mythical sea monster Leviathan and beast Behemoth or "learn to extol an existence in which chaos is a real and threatening force."[85]

The theophany is not a rational or logical discourse. God appears in a whirlwind to expose Job to a multitude of rhetorical questions and imperatives:

> Who is this that darkens counsel by words without knowledge?
> Gird up your loins like a man,
>     I will question you, and you shall declare to me.
> Where were you when I laid the foundation of the earth?
> Tell me, if you have understanding (Job 38:2-4).

Poet Job continues in a cadence of rhetorical questions to form a ground swell of rhythmic melody to instill a subliminal message which forces Job to let go of all his preconceived images, metaphors and models of God.

The powers of human imagination expose the theological creativity of Poet Job to reach out through the window of vulnerability toward God. The theophany (Job 38:1–42:6) asks humanity:

> Have you commanded the morning since your days began?
>     (Job 38:12).

> Have you entered the storehouses of the snow? (Job 38:22).

> Has the rain a father,
>     or who has begotten the drops of dew?
> From whose womb did the ice come forth,
>     and who has given birth to the hoarfrost of heaven?
>         (Job 38:28-29)

> Can you lift your voice to the clouds,
>     so that a flood of waters may cover you?
> Can you send forth lightnings, so that they may go
>     and say to you, 'Here we are'?
> Who has put wisdom in the inward parts,
>     or given understanding to the mind? (Job 38:34-36).

> Do you know when the mountain goats give birth?
>     Do you observe the calving of the deer? . . .
> Who has let the wild ass go free? . . .

> Is the wild ox willing to serve you?
>     Will it spend the night at your crib? . . .
> Is it by your wisdom that the hawk soars,
>     and spreads its wings toward the south? (Job 39:1, 5, 9, 26).

Job and the reader, you and I, become sensually transformed
as we are invited to approach a primal energy independent of
human thought and feeling. We are transported toward the
elemental reality of the indestructible power and indestructible
joy innate to the creation. And with this movement, there
comes an acceptance that the cosmos is very good even though
pain and suffering exist within it.

Now rationality and pragmatism do not have the final
word. In Job's spiritual awakening the manifestation and mystery of God appear to stand in a theological paradox with pain
and suffering. This is a world of which God was able to say:
"God saw everything that he had made, and indeed it was very
good" (Gen 1:31).

Women and men may prefer a world-picture dominated by
doctrines and dogma, rationality and reason, science and pragmatic piety, because these provide a stable, predictable, con-
trollable world-view. Poet Job, however, challenges us to accept
the frightening and fascinating theocentric world of ecological
interdependence, relationship and encounter in which epiphany occurs.

Poet Job shares with the reader the daring, countercultural
theology of a God in relationship and communication with humanity. Job becomes the prophet who flings open the door and
presents the paradox of a theology of emotional experience of
the sacred and the magnificent mystery of God.

Job's theology denies an omnipotent, distant, retribution-
seeking God of the moral order, while it nonetheless acknowledges the power of God in creation. Job's spirituality is awake
and he has opened the window of vulnerability for all of humanity to step through. Job asks us to share the light of the in-
breaking of God in our times of trouble and tragedy.

# Reflection

The priest placed the sacramental stole around her neck. The colors of God's promise to humanity brought light into the room. The purple of iris on a winter's day, the bright blue of a hot summer's day, the green of verdant hills after winter rains, the yellow of the harvest moon and the white of driven snow— all were quilted together in a Seminole Indian Patchwork pattern and bound within a border of brightest red.

I remembered the journey I had taken to find just the right silk fabrics to make this stole. What had started out as a day of frustration became an experience of epiphany. It happened on Good Friday. As I was driving down the coast road, the vista of Sea greeting Land was a powerful sign for me to stop driving and listen.

I parked my Honda and, sitting down on the promontory, I began to read the Liturgy for Good Friday. I meditated on the Gospel account of the Crucifixion, read the psalms, "My God, my God, why have you forsaken me?" (Psalm 22:1), and read the collects for the creation and our needs.

I meditated as I watched the depth of the sea; smooth to the eye but powerful in life-giving and life-taking. The waters were changed as they reached the land; the projection of hard rock on the margins changed the flow of water across the incoming waves. Waves which came in beyond the margins crashed in thunder, foam and chaos; the cross waves joined the incoming waves beyond the promontory and gently eased upon a sandy beach in multiple fingers stretched upon Earth, only to be rapidly reclaimed by the ever changing water of Sea.

I returned to my car and sped across the asphalt toward my goal. But I remembered a pathway across the foothills of the peninsula; it was a day for wandering and erring. I lost my way, found my way into a small town called Honda, passed the beauty of woodlands and the spring flowers; I was passed in

leaps and bounds of freedom by a deer as she crashed through
the hedge onto the road in front of my car.

I stopped to pick a few forget-me-nots growing in abundance
by the roadside; "Why have you forsaken me?" I put the flowers
in the shade on the floor of my car. I reached my destination,
brought the vibrant threads from the Silkworm and headed
home in the traffic and congestion of a late Friday afternoon.

On the third day I was up early before the skirts of dawn
were shaken. The light of Christ broke the darkness. After
celebration, conversation and carnival in community I drove
home. On the floor of my car I saw the flowers I had picked Friday, now shriveled and lifeless. I had taken them in their beauty
of life and strength and now they lay forgotten. I picked them
up and placed them in a dish, now empty of the food I had
taken to the communal breakfast.

Later on Sunday I joined friends for supper. On walking up
the cold, concrete stairs I found my neglected forget-me-nots.
Humbly I bent to pick them up again and took them to my
room. I am not sure why but I put them gently into a vase of
dried flowers by my sink and poured water into the vase and
sprinkled them. The next morning the dried brown leaves of
the past three days were scarred but green. The drooping, lifeless blue and yellow heads of yesterday were wondrously vibrant and upright.

My reverie was broken when the priest called upon the
saints to be present as holy water was sprinkled into each nook
and cranny of the room and called upon God's steadfast love
to be present. Slowly the chrism was applied to limbs which we
had constantly bathed with ointments to relieve the travesty of
psoriasis. The oil soothed the limbs where once invisible bones,
gnawed by pain, now thrust themselves into conflict with the
skin to deny it life and rot the flesh. The words of unction
reached the dying and smiles crossed the faces in the room.

Peace entered that troubled room. Grace was present when
a weak hand searched for forehead, chest, right breast, left
breast and returned to the center. By touch a ring was removed

and given to a life-partner. Life ebbed away but in the dying moment hands reached up to God. The morning stars sang together and the shouts of joy were heard as the skirts of dawn were shaken that day.

I know God cares for my spirit, always.

———————

At the start of the theophany, Job has become the hero of defiance for all of humanity's suffering. He has thrown out the friends' explanations of the community's traditional views of a theology of retribution. He has demanded to see his God, face to face.

Job believes in the radical concept of a God in relationship and communication with humanity.

The answers Job sought on behalf of all of humanity are given to him through a paradoxical covenanting convergence.

Having let go of his need for rational answers, Job exists in a place of vulnerability which makes it possible for him to move into a spiritual encounter with God.

The center of the poet's work shifts in the theophany from the rationality of moral human righteousness and legalism to the beauty of an inner peace and awareness of the awesome nature of the world around us.

In the end, there are no rational answers to the question of pain and suffering.

Pain and suffering are neither condoned nor explained.

All that occurs is a presentation of creation and relationship with a God who cares for our spirits.

Poet Job's world-picture requires a world of meaning wherein risk and paradox exist and where a willingness to accept essential and indissoluble contradictions acknowledges human vulnerability.

# − 8 −

# Epilogue

The child sits amidst a stand of trees. These are no ordinary trees but the giant Redwood trees of Muir Woods. A tree towering tall and timeless spreads a dome of green above her; sunlight shines through the clerestory branches in the dark shield above to flash upon a deer nonchalantly munching sweet grass just a few steps away.

The overpowering darkness and silence appear to paralyze the child's speech and movement. She sits so still. She stays like this, isolated from her companions. The sunlight plays on her yellow dress. Gradually her eyes become accustomed to the impartial dimness. She becomes aware of the smell of moss, mold and compost.

The fragile ferns acquire identity to stand, svelte guardians over the tiniest of plants and this fragile being. She does not know their names, nor does she wish to name or own them. The familiar universality of their essence in the form of daisy, bell and trumpet, stalk and leaf, praise the God who made the intricate life of the universal forest stretched around, beneath, within her.

In growing awareness the distinctive, naming redness of the Redwood is no longer red but multi-shades of brown, gray, brightest orange, cinnamon and crimson touched with ocher, green and black—to name but just a few; the naming colors of diversity glimmer through the multifaceted shades of an impartial darkness.

The trees obscure the light but form a whole where grounded beginnings and top-most branches are only obscured by the child's stance. The tree's beginnings are deep, deep beneath her in the rich nitrous soil of loss and death; its top-most branches live in freedom reaching far for light, for moisture and for warmth. The tree's branches tip their graceful ends toward the nurturing sky above, seeking growth and life.

On close inspection the friendly tree is itself a thoroughfare of life. The tangled web of branches make a suburban community where ants and beetles make their tenuous homes; homes where they become the prey of transient butterflies, of sparrows, of jaunty tits and raucous jays. Unnamed, acrobatic squirrels, on their daily travels, launch themselves in space toward the branches of the Redwood tree and drop their acorns as gentle gifts to the girl below.

Quietly she stretches out her hand to pick up her gift; slowly she stands amongst the Redwood trees and realizes the sun is setting. Soon the heavenly beings will shout for joy as the swaddling bands of darkness envelope a world where she is one of the millions of people who daily face tragedy: she has AIDS.

# Appendix

## Outline of *Job* Juxtaposed with Stages of Suffering

| | |
|---|---|
| Prose prologue | Job 1–2:13 |
| **Silence on the dung heap**<br>*First stage of suffering: Mute* | Job 2:13 |
| **Conversation**<br>*Second stage of suffering: Expressive* | Job 3–42:6 |
| First cycle | Job 3–14 |
| Second cycle | Job 15–21 |
| Third cycle | Job 22–27 |
| Wisdom Hymn | Job 28 |
| Job sums up | Job 29–31 |
| Fourth friend | Job 32–37 |
| Voice of the Lord | Job 38–41 |
| Job's final answer | Job 42:1-6 |
| **Prose epilogue**<br>*Third stage of suffering: Change Incorporated* | Job 42:7-17 |

# Bibliography

Achtemeier, Paul J., gen. ed. *Harper's Bible Dictionary*. San Francisco: Harper and Row, Publishers, 1985.

Andersen, Francis. *Job: An Introduction and Commentary*. Leicester: Inter-Varsity Press, 1976.

Brueggemann, Walter. *The Message of the Psalms: A Theological Commentary*. Minneapolis: Augsberg Press, 1984.

Chaisson, Eric. *Cosmic Dawn*. Boston: Little, Brown and Company, 1981.

Cowan, Georgianne. "The Sacred Womb." *The Soul of Nature: Visions of a Living Earth*. Ed. Michael Tobias and Georgianne Cowan. New York: Continuum, 1994.

Craven, Tony. *The Book of Psalms*. Message of Biblical Spirituality. Collegeville: The Liturgical Press, 1992.

Davis, Ellen F. "Job and Jacob: The Integrity of Faith." *Reading Between the Texts: Intertextuality and the Hebrew Bible*. Ed. Danna Nolan Fewell. Louisville: John Knox Press, 1992.

Entretien, Xlle. "Cours Familier de Literature" (Paris, 1955) II, 441. Trans. Evelyn Simha, in *Dimensions of Job: A Study and Selected Readings*. Ed. Nahum Glatzer. New York: Schoken, 1969.

Fohrer, George. *Man and Disease According to the Book of Job* in "Koroth," vol. 9. Proceedings of the International Symposium on Medicine in Bible and Talmud. Jerusalem: Menahem Press, 1987.

Genova, Judith. *Wittgenstein: A Way of Seeing*. New York: Routledge, 1995.

Gergen, Kenneth J. *The Saturated Self: Dilemmas of Identity in Contemporary Life*. San Francisco: Harper Collins, 1991.

Gordis, Robert. *The Book of Job: Commentary, New York Translation and Special Studies.* New York: Jewish Theological Seminary of America, 1978.

Griffen, David Ray. "Introduction." *Spirituality and Society.* Ed. David Ray Griffen. New York: State University of New York Press, 1988.

Habel, Norman C. *The Book of Job: A Commentary.* The Old Testament Library. Philadelphia: The Westminster Press, 1985.

Hoffman, Yair. "Irony in the Book of Job." *Immanuel: A Bulletin of Religious Thought and Research in Israel* (No. 17, Winter 1983/84) Jerusalem: The Ecumenical Theological Research Fraternity in Israel.

Janzen, Gerald J. *Job.* Interpretation: A Biblical Commentary for Teaching and Preaching. Atlanta: John Knox, 1990.

Kubler-Ross, Elisabeth. *On Death and Dying.* New York: Macmillan Company, 1969.

_____. *AIDS: The Ultimate Challenge.* New York: Macmillan Company, 1987.

Kushner, Harold S. *When Bad Things Happen to Good People.* Avon Books. New York: The Hearst Corporation, 1981.

Levin, Simon S. *Adam's Rib: Essays on Biblical Medicine.* Los Altos: Geron-X, Inc., 1970.

Loewy, Erich H. *Suffering and the Beneficent Community: Beyond Libertarianism.* New York: State University Press, 1991.

May, Herbert G., and Bruce M. Metzer. *The New Oxford Annotated Bible, RSV.* New York: Oxford University Press, 1991.

McFague, Sallie. *Models of God: Theology for an Ecological, Nuclear Age.* Philadelphia: Fortress Press, 1987.

Mitchell, Stephen. *The Book of Job.* San Francisco: North Point Press, 1987.

Murphy, Roland E. *The Tree of Life: An Exploration of Biblical Wisdom Literature.* The Anchor Bible Reference Library. New York: Doubleday, 1990.

National Commission on AIDS. *AIDS: An Expanding Tragedy.* June E. Osborn, Chairman. Washington, D.C., 1993.

Penchansky, David. *The Betrayal of God: Ideological Conflict in Job.* Louisville: Westminster/John Knox Press, 1990.

Perdue, Leo. *Wisdom in Revolt: Metaphorical Theology in the Book of Job.* Sheffield: The Almond Press, 1991.

_____. *Wisdom and Creation: The Theology of Wisdom Literature.* Nashville: Abingdon Press, 1994.

Perdue, Leo, and W. Clark Gilpen, eds. *The Voice from the Whirlwind: Interpreting the Book of Job.* Nashville: Abingdon Press, 1992.

Pritchard, James B., ed. *The Ancient Near East,* vol. 2. Princeton: Princeton University Press, 1975.

Robinson, Gene. "Hope for Uganda." *The Drum.* Ed. Albert J. Ogle (Winter, 1992) Pasadena: Uganda AIDS Project.

Soelle, Dorothee. *Suffering.* Trans. Everett R. Kalin. Philadelphia: Fortress Press, 1973.

_____. *The Window of Vulnerability.* Trans. Linda M. Maloney. Minneapolis: Fortress Press, 1990.

Sontag, Susan. *AIDS and Its Metaphors.* New York: Farrar, Straus and Giroux, 1988.

Stadelman, S.J., Luis. *The Hebrew Conception of the World: A Philological and Literary Study.* Rome: Pontifical Biblical Institute, 1970.

Tillich, Paul. *The Meaning of Health.* Ed. Paul Lee. Richmond, Calif.: North Atlantic Books, 1981.

Toorn, K. van der. *Sin and Sanction in Israel and Mesopotamia.* The Netherlands: Van Gorcum, 1985.

Touraine, Alain. *Critique of Modernity.* Oxford, U.K. and Cambridge, U.S.A.: Blackwell, 1995.

# Notes

1. *AIDS an Expanding Tragedy,* National Commission on AIDS (Washington, 1993) vii.

2. Both the Vulgate and Septuagint translations of Job 2:8 use *dung heap* for *ashes* in the phrase "and sat among the ashes."

3. Gene Robinson, "Hope for Uganda," *The Drum* (Winter, 1992) 1.

4. The dating of *Job* as a sophisticated literary product ranges from the tenth to the fourth century B.C.E. with most evidence pointing to the text being written in the post-exilic era (fourth century B.C.E.) I concur with this dating.

5. Gerald J. Janzen, *Job,* Interpretation, A Bible Commentary for Teaching and Preaching (Atlanta: John Knox, 1990) 4.

6. Harold S. Krushner, *When Bad Things Happen to Good People* (New York: Avon Books, 1981) 134.

7. Simon S. Levin, *Adam's Rib* (Los Altos: Geron-X, Inc., 1970) 79–80.

8. K. Van der Toorn, *Sin and Sanction in Israel and Mesopotamia* (The Netherlands: Van Gorcum, 1985) 71–76.

9. Xlle. Entretien, "Cours Familier de Literature," translated by Evelyn Simha in *Dimensions of Job: A Study and Selected Readings,* ed., Nahum N. Glatzer (New York: Schoken, 1969) 43.

10. Norman C. Habel, *The Book of Job: A Commentary* (Philadelphia: The Westminster Press, 1985) 391.

11. Ibid., 392.

12. Ibid., 394.

13. Ibid., 423–24.

14. Ibid., 4.

15. Yair Hoffman, "Irony in the Book of Job," *Immanuel* (No. 17, Winter, 1983/84) 7.

16. James B. Pritchard, ed., *The Ancient Near East: A New Anthology of Texts and Pictures* (Princeton: Princeton University Press, 1975) 136–41, 160–67.

17. Ibid., 160–61.

18. Ibid., 139.

19. Eliphaz and Teman both appear in Edomite genealogies. Shuhite is probably linked to Shuah, a son of Abraham by Keturah. Naamahite derives from Naamah, a female descendent of Cain (Habel, *The Book of Job*, 97).

20. The three friends follow the traditional consoling role of a friend in ancient society. They weep, tear their clothes and fling dust upon their heads in total empathy with Job. (Ibid.).

21. Ibid., 13.

22. Janzen, *Job*, 20–21.

23. Luis Stadelmann, S.J., *The Hebrew Conception of the World: A Philological and Literary Study*, (Rome: Pontifical Biblical Institute, 1970) 10–13.

24. Leo Perdue, *Wisdom and Creation* (Nashville: Abingdon Press, 1994) 134.

25. Perdue, *Wisdom in Revolt* (Sheffield: The Almond Press, 1991) 74.

26. Janzen, *Job*, 5. Although Janzen writes from the premise that *Job* was written in the Exile this point is also valid for a post-exilic writer.

27. Ibid., 5.

28. Ibid., 5–7.

29. Ibid., 8.

30. Ibid., 8.

31. Ibid., 8–10.

32. Ibid., 10.

33. Habel, *The Book of Job*, 42.

34. Judith Genova, *Wittgenstein: A Way of Seeing* (New York: Routledge, 1955) 51.

35. Georgianne Cowan, "The Sacred Womb," in *The Soul of Nature*, ed. Michael Tobies and Georgianne Cowan (New York: Continuum, 1994) 139.

36. David Ray Griffen, ed. *Spirituality and Society: Postmodern Visions* (New York: State University of New York Press, 1988) 1.

37. Susan Sontag's *AIDS and Its Metaphors* is very helpful in explaining how the language used for disease shapes our perception and, frequently, our response.

38. Leo Purdue provides multiple references for the study of metaphor in religion in his book, *Wisdom in Revolt: Metaphorical Theology for the Book of Job*, 22.

39. Perdue, *Wisdom in Revolt*, 5.

40. Sallie McFague, *Models of God* (Philadelphia: Fortress Press, 1987) 34.

41. Eric Chaisson, *Cosmic Dawn* (Boston: Little, Brown and Company, 1981) 40.

42. Ibid., 42.

43. Ibid., 126.

44. Ibid., 77.

45. Ibid., 52.

46. Kenneth J. Gergen, *The Saturated Self* (San Francisco: Harper Collins, 1991) 6.

47. Stadelmann, *The Hebrew Conception of the World*, 26–28.

48. Alain Touraine, *Critique of Modernity* (Oxford, UK and Cambridge, U.S.A., 1995) 29–47.

49. Gustafson, "A Response to the Book of Job," *The Voice from the Whirlwind*, Leo Purdue and W. Clark Gilpen, eds. (Nashville: Abingdon Press, 1992) 180.

50. Kushner, *When Bad Things Happen to Good People*, 134.

51. Perdue, *Wisdom and Creation*, 174.

52. Many years ago a patient had a stuffed rabbit she named Damn-It. Now I meet patients and friends who own "Damn-It Dolls" which they claim are designed for venting frustrations.

53. Perdue, *Wisdom and Creation*, 30.

54. Dorothee Soelle, *The Window of Vulnerability* (Minneapolis: Fortress Press, 1990) viii.

55. Susan Sontag, *AIDS and Its Metaphors* (New York: Farrar, Straus and Giroux, 1988) 94.

56. Soelle, *The Window of Vulnerability*, ix.

57. Ibid., x.

58. Janzen, *Job*, 35.

59. Ellen F. Davis, "Job and Jacob: The Integrity of Faith," *Reading Between the Texts*, ed. Danna Nolan Fewell (Louisville: John Knox Press, 1992) 204.

60. Paul Tillich, *The Meaning of Health* (Richmond, Calif.: North Atlantic Books, 1981) 51.

61. Ibid., 53.

62. A random, unscientific survey among women friends revealed an immediate acknowledgment of this as an unrecognized but real experience of suffering.

63. Erich H. Loewy, *Suffering and the Beneficent Community* (New York: State University Press, 1991) 5–6.

64. Habel, *The Book of Job*, 148.

65. Ibid., 148.

66. Dorothee Soelle, *Suffering* (Philadelphia: Fortress Press, 1973) 73.

67. Ibid., 70–74.

68. Elizabeth Kubler-Ross, *AIDS: The Ultimate Challenge* (New York: Macmillan Company, 1987) 1–2.

69. Tony Craven, *The Book of Psalms* (Collegeville: The Liturgical Press, 1992) 49.

70. The sacred curse was a common practice in biblical times. An individual or a magician made a pronouncement upon an enemy or person suspected of a crime. It was understood, however, that the curse only went into effect if a person was indeed guilty. The craft of the magician was to be able to effectively pull together either evil or positive powers to influence human life. The religious Israelite lived within this ethos but also believed Yahweh was, ultimately, in control. In serious situations petition was made to God for justice, for the Israelites understood that vengeance belonged to God alone.

71. Janzen, *Job*, 62.

72. The accepted sequence for the lament of an individual in the psalms is: address, lament/complaint, confession of trust, petition, assurance of being heard and vow of praise (Craven, *Book of Psalms*, 27). Walter Brueggemann describes the lament psalms as "poems of disorientation" for the seasons of hurt, alienation, suffering and death. See Brueggemann's *The Message of the Psalms* (Minneapolis: Augsberg Press, 1984) 19.

73. Janzen, *Job*, 66: "trouble"; Habel, *The Book of Job* 112: "turmoil."

74. Habel, *The Book of Job*, 157.

75. Janzen, *Job*, 81; Habel, *The Book of Job*, 157.

76. Habel, *The Book of Job*, 162.

77. Ibid., 155.

78. Ibid., 209.

79. Robert Gordis, *The Book of Job* (New York: Jewish Theological Seminary of America, 1978) 526–35.

80. Soren Kierkegaard, "Repetitions," *The Tree of Life,* ed. Roland E. Murphy (New York: Doubleday, 1990) 38–39.

81. Stadelmann, *The Hebrew Conception of the World,* 101.

82. Literary analysis for the theophany is taken from Perdue's *Wisdom in Revolt.*

83. "The horse was first domesticated in the Eurasian steppes, probably around 3000 B.C.E. . . . (and) introduced into Palestine by the Hykos in the first half of the second millennium B.C.E." Paul J. Achtemeier, gen. ed. *Harper's Bible Dictionary* (San Francisco: Harper and Row Publishers, 1985) 406.

84. Stephen Mitchell, *The Book of Job* (San Francisco: North Point Press, 1987) xx.

85. Perdue, *Wisdom in Revolt,* 221.